Living Lite

Ultra Low-Fat & Fat-Free Recipes

Original recipes devised by

Sandy Frazer

Living Lite

Published by Cut & Paste Studio Pty Ltd
ABN 57 090 761 710
39 First Avenue Bridgewater SA 5155 Australia
Enquiries: Contact Living Lite (08) 8339 4536
Email: livlite@hotmail.com

1st printing: 2000
2nd printing: 2001

ISBN 0-646-40329-X

The information in this book is not intended as a substitute for consulting
with your physician or other health care provider. The publisher and
author are not responsible for any adverse effects or consequences
resulting from the use of any suggestions, preparations or procedures
contained in this book. All matters relating to your health should be
discussed with your doctor.

Printed and bound by Hyde Park Press
4 Deacon Avenue, Richmond SA 5033

Cover, book design & photography by Cut & Paste Studio Pty Ltd

All recipes in this book were analysed using the nutrition information
provided on the product labels.

Living Lite

Ultra Low-Fat & Fat-Free Recipes

Acknowledgements

The following people enrich my life daily. Without them this book would never have eventuated.

My husband Paul, lover and best friend - we continue to share the same dreams and ambitions. Changing our lifestyle 8 years ago was just another of the many things we have done together. Your never-ending patience and tolerance, positive energy, motivation, persistence and your brilliant photos and cover design, have made this project a very special joint venture.

Ben, our son - you have tried and tasted so many of my cooking experiments. Your patience and your eternal tolerance of your busy parents' lives, is unbelievable. Continue to be healthy!

Mum & Dad - thank you for your continual understanding, encouragement and support - and for being gourmet guinea pigs! Thank you also for your meticulous proofreading.

Elda & Fred Frazer, my parents-in-law - you have always taken great interest in the progress of my book and given wonderful support and understanding in our preferred lifestyle.

The rest of our family on both sides - you may be amused at our fussy eating sometimes, but you all take our lifestyle seriously. You continually put yourselves out to provide suitable food, and are not offended when we bring our own! Thank you.

Our wonderful group of special friends who care enough to design their dinner party menus around us! - You know who you are. Your tireless efforts, thoughtfulness and consideration are truly appreciated. You have also been suspecting (and unsuspecting) guinea pigs! To the many of you who encouraged me to write this book, and have continually enquired on its progress for as long as it has taken, I thank you.

Contents

Introduction

The low-fat recipes in *Living Lite* are just some of the many I have devised since realising that following a low-fat lifestyle is the only way to lose fat - and keep it off. It is certainly how I managed to lose my excess 30kg, and my husband, his excess 20kg. By "Living Lite" we have both kept it off and have successfully maintained our ideal body weight for over eight years.

In 1992, I was very unhappy with the way I looked and felt. I was fast outgrowing size 16 clothes, and climbing just one small flight of stairs left me short of breath. I had lost weight numerous times in the past only to regain it. I knew the yo-yo dieting had to stop and if I wanted permanent results, I had to do it properly. I also realised it was *fat* I needed to lose, not just weight. It was easy to identify the problem - I was fat because I *consumed* too much fat, which meant more calories than I was burning off!

By eliminating all added fat from my diet and walking for 20 minutes every day, the weight just fell off - not quickly, but gradually and naturally. I knew I had reached my goal the day I was able to easily slip into a size 10 pair of jeans! Eight years later, they still fit me.

Anybody can lose weight, but the only way to keep it off permanently is to modify one's eating habits and follow a low-fat lifestyle that incorporates interesting and regular exercise. I know most people think that eating low-fat means giving up flavour. The recipes in this book will show you otherwise. You will see that by using clever, simple techniques and substitutions for high fat ingredients, you can eat virtually anything - from laksas to chocolate cake. Low-fat eating does not mean having to give up sweet creamy desserts or cakes. I've devised hundreds of low-fat sweet recipes that prove you can eat these and still stay slim. I'm astounded at how often I've heard someone who is trying to trim down, proudly boast that they've eaten nothing all day! You cannot lose weight successfully by severely restricting the volume of food you consume. I eat more food now than I did when I was overweight - but now I eat the way the food is prepared in *Living Lite*.

Reading and understanding food labels is essential in successfully eliminating excess fat. Most people are totally unaware of how much hidden fat is contained in commercial food products. I quickly learnt to ignore many manufacturers' product claims. Study the labels properly and you will find many "lite" products are pumped up with extra sugar to compensate for the lower fat content. Some serve sizes are also smaller than their original full-fat version and actually contain more calories than the original version! However, there are some excellent low-fat and fat-free products on the market. Each time you reach for a product, stop to check other product labels for a low-fat or fat-free alternative. I find new products and ingredients all the time that are suitable for use in this method of cooking. Australia has an abundance of fabulous ingredients available from which you can create all sorts of low-fat delicious dishes.

This lifestyle is second nature to us, a way of life. We never feel we're missing out or deprived. If we feel like a certain food, we simply modify. I could never imagine returning to our former eating habits. Living this way has meant we have never regained our weight.

I spend the majority of my spare time writing recipes, cooking and experimenting with new food combinations and on most days, come up with four or five new recipes. This means I'm often up at 5am. I have written *Living Lite* to share the results of these experiments (and early mornings!) with you.

I would love any feedback about *Living Lite*. Maybe you have a question, information or a request for future recipe inclusion as *Living Lite 2* is already under way (see page 155) You may wish to send me a favourite recipe that I can attempt to "low-fat modify" for you. Please include a stamped self-addressed envelope for reply. You can write to me at:

39 First Avenue, Bridgewater SA 5155
   or
Email: livlite@hotmail.com
   or
Fax: (08) 8339 8224

Living Lite means:

Limiting your fat intake to 20% of your daily calorie intake
This means around 45-50 grams for the average woman and around
60 grams for the average man. To lose weight, aim for around 15-20
grams. Some Australians eat 50% of their intake in fat and it is not
difficult to consume this much - one takeaway hamburger can
contain 40 grams of fat! Every fat gram contains 9 calories, whereas
carbohydrates and proteins carry only 4 calories per gram. Some fat
is necessary as it provides essential fatty acids and fat-soluble
vitamins A, D and E. It is impossible to eat no fat even if eating "fat-
free".
Conditions associated with eating too much fat are heart disease,
diabetes, some cancers, gallstones, obesity, high blood pressure and
high cholesterol levels.

Eating a wide variety of foods.
By eating a wide variety of textures, colours, tastes, even
temperatures you will feel more satisfied. Increase your intake of
fruits and vegetables for filling, low-fat satisfaction. Make them a part
of every meal.

Eating between meals
This is important. Don't sit down to every meal ravenously hungry.
But make sure your snacks are healthy – fresh or dried fruit,
complex carbohydrates, low-fat cakes etc. Don't believe that if you
are feeling hungry you are losing weight - it is actually having the
opposite effect on your body. The hungrier you let yourself feel, the
more fat your body holds onto.

Eating slowly
It takes 20 minutes for your brain to register you are full. Give the
brain time to work, and eat in a relaxed state.

Drinking lots of water
Aim for 6-8 glasses a day. We are often thirsty when we think we are
hungry. Afternoon slumps in energy are often a sign of dehydration.

Slenderising your kitchen

There are low-fat versions of many foods on the market. And there are hundreds of naturally low-fat foods available. Buy lots of herbs and spices. Don't fry in oil. Prepare food by grilling, baking, poaching, dry-frying, steaming, microwaving, and sautéing in wine, stock, water, vinegar or lemon juice. See pages 7-9 and 141-144 for more information on "slenderising" your kitchen.

Performing aerobic & anaerobic exercise

Aerobic - Aim for at least 20 minutes 3 times a week. This includes walking, swimming, cycling.
Anaerobic - Aim for 20 minutes 3 times a week. This is weight training and resistance training. Join a gym or do this at home with free weights. Remember that the calories and fat you consume are burned by *muscle tissue*. Muscle burns fat.
Exercise is important for longevity, stress relief, energy increase. It increases your metabolism, lowers cholesterol and fights fat. Exercise suppresses appetite - it doesn't increase it. Research has shown that the harder you exercise, the longer your appetite is lowered. Just a little exercise is better than none at all.

Stress management

Get sleep, relaxation and time out. And exercise! Exercise reduces stress.

Smart shopping

Read labels and learn to understand nutritional panels. Analyse the *fat percentage per 100 calories* not percentage per 100g weight. Aim for no more than 2 grams of fat in every 100 calories. This means only 18% of the calorie intake is fat. See page 7 for more information on "Smart Shopping".

Realising the difference between appetite and hunger

Appetite stems from the brain, but hunger stems from the stomach.

Giving it a go!

This is the most important. In 30 days Living Lite can become a lifestyle. Think "Living Lite" all day, every day.

The less fat you eat, the less fat you crave!

Smart Shopping

Living Lite begins with a healthy shopping trolley.

♥ Avoid food shopping when you're hungry. You'll be more easily tempted to make high-fat purchases.

♥ Fill your supermarket trolley with fresh fruit and vegetables before moving on to other sections of the supermarket.

♥ Select breads that have at least 2g fibre per serve.

♥ Give yourself time to read the labels and learn which products are better choices.

♥ Check the fat information on the nutrition label. Labelling laws mean there's no excuse for not reducing your fat intake.

♥ Don't always rely on "fat-free" claims on packaging – more often than not, they contain extra sugar to compensate.

♥ Foods with labels that state no cholesterol can still be filled with fat.

♥ Check serving sizes – some are very unrealistic.

♥ Buy plain frozen vegetables, not varieties with sauces included –they can contain up to an extra 7 grams of fat per serving.

♥ Buy tuna packed in springwater, not oil, and save 8 grams of fat per 185g can.

♥ Buy lean cuts of meat, chicken and fish instead of fatty, marbled varieties.

♥ Avoid pre-crumbed foods (they usually have added fat) and crumb your own instead.

♥ If you are time-poor, buy the prepacked shredded and chopped vegetables to whip up a quick stir-fry or salad.

♥ Buy fat-free dressings, sauces, mustards and vinegars for boosting the flavour in your cooking.

♥ Buy canned fruit packed in natural juice not syrup.

♥ Choose fat-free and skim varieties of dairy – they still contain the calcium, protein and vitamins.

♥ Avoid rich ice creams – they are loaded with fat.

♥ Buy water ice blocks not chocolate creamy iced treats.

The Living Lite Pantry

Fill your fat-free pantry with these food items and you should be able to prepare a low-fat healthy meal quickly and easily. Check the label for oil or fat listings.

Fresh - fruits and vegetables in season, onions, carrots, celery, potatoes, mushrooms, lemons, limes

Frozen - fruits and vegetables, chicken breast fillets, lean meats

Dairy - "fat-free", "low-fat" and "skim" products - milk, yoghurts (fruit & plain), cottage cheese, ricotta cheese, Parmesan, evaporated low-fat milk, milk powder, and low-fat ice cream

Bottled - garlic, ginger, chilli paste, lemongrass, horseradish

Jars - tomato paste, relishes, pickles, gherkins, pickled onions,

Cans - vegetables, beans, chickpeas, tuna, salmon, sweet corn, pie apples for making apple puree, tomatoes, tomato puree, fruit (in water or unsweetened juice)

Fat-free sauces - hoisin, tomato, teriyaki, barbecue, sweet chilli, chilli, Worcestershire, HP, steak, plum, Tabasco, liquid smoke, low-salt soy, assorted mustards - dijon, seeded, German, tarragon

Fat-free dressings and mayonnaise - French, Italian, honey & mustard, Greek, balsamic

Dried fruits - sultanas, dates, apricots, figs, currants, sun-dried tomatoes

Vinegars - balsamic, white, cider, white wine, red wine, tarragon

Egg-free pasta - penne, fettucine, spaghetti, couscous

Rice - basmati, jasmine, brown, arborio

Bread & biscuits - low-fat breads, 98% fat-free Salada, rice cakes, pita bread, fat-free croutons, pretzels, rice crackers

Cereals - oats, processed and unprocessed bran, Nutrigrain, low-fat muesli

Flours - plain & self-raising, wholemeal, white, cornflour

Baking products - essences, breadcrumbs, cornflake crumbs, cocoa powder, baking powder, bicarb of soda, yeast, non-stick spray, gelatine, Splenda, egg substitute powder, eggs for whites, honey, prune puree, apple juice concentrate, corn syrup, rice syrup, maple syrup, low-joule jelly crystals

Dried herbs and spices - stock powders, salt, pepper, oregano, Italian, basil, parsley, onion powder, garlic powder, cumin, cinnamon, coriander, paprika, bay leaves, chilli powder, ginger, nutmeg, onion flakes, rosemary, thyme, tarragon

Miscellaneous - low-joule toppings, jams (no added sugar)

Fat-Free Meal Production

1. Invest in good quality non-stick cookware. It can be expensive to buy but it is worth the cost and will last for a long time. You will need cooking pots and pans, assorted shaped cake tins, muffin pans, a wok, and a fry pan. Use only wooden or plastic utensils to avoid scratching them. I have found *Bakers Secret* to be the best quality non-stick baking cookware on the market.

2. Buy baking paper. Can be used on all cake pans, oven trays, for cooking in frying pans and even to line the sandwich maker. It saves on cleaning, it protects the cookware and means cooking requires NO FAT!

3. A microwave is invaluable. It can create and reheat quick, healthy meals in minutes. You can purchase a small microwave for the price of 2 meals eaten out!

4. A food processor and a blender are two appliances I could not do without. I use them all the time for pureeing soups, fruits, sauces, dressings, dips and making smoothies. They are also wonderful time savers for when you need to do large amounts of grating and chopping. A hand held blender (like a Bamix) is also very handy.

5. Every kitchen needs measuring equipment i.e. Metric measuring spoons and cups. I find kitchen scales for accurate weight measurements a necessity. Also, an assortment of whisks and glass baking dishes.

6. Luxuries that I am lucky enough to own, but are not essential include a bread maker, an ice cream maker and a juicer.

For your Information:

1. Ingredients in the recipes marked with * are described in the glossary (see page 147). Where to buy them is also included. Unusual ingredients are available in Asian stores and health food stores, however supermarkets now are beginning to carry an enormous range of foods.

2. Oven temperatures are for fan-forced ovens. Please refer to your oven manual for temperature adjustments.

3. All measurements are Australian standard.
   1 tablespoon = 20 mls   1 cup = 250mls

4. Foods listed below are high in fat and not used in this book. For "Living Lite", limit their intake (or better still, eliminate.)
   - Egg yolks - the whites contain no fat
   - Hard cheeses – I use 1 tbspn Parmesan for flavour in an entire dish only adding about 3g fat.
   - All oils, butter, margarine, ghee, lard, copha, solid frying vegetable oil
   - All full cream dairy products – buy "skim" and "non-fat"
   - Commercial biscuits, cakes, pies and pastry bases
   - Nuts & seeds - limited amounts are used – good for you but consume in moderation as they are high in fat
   - Traditional commercial mayonnaises and dressings – contain oil and egg yolk
   - Olives, coconuts and avocadoes – high in fat.
     Use small amounts and use in moderation
   - Smallgoods – salami, metwurst, polish sausage etc
   - Solid chocolate – cocoa butter is what sets chocolate

5. Fat calculations in chicken recipes were made using Steggles chicken breast fillets. The fat in Steggles breast fillets is only ·6 per 100g.

6. As with all recipes, it is always a good idea to read through the entire recipe before starting to ensure you have everything required on hand.

7. As most households have a microwave oven, some of the recipes are microwave prepared. If you don't have a microwave oven, these recipes can quite easily be cooked conventionally.

Living Lite

soups

Photo right: *Spiced Bean, Pasta & Tomato Soup*
(recipe page 18)

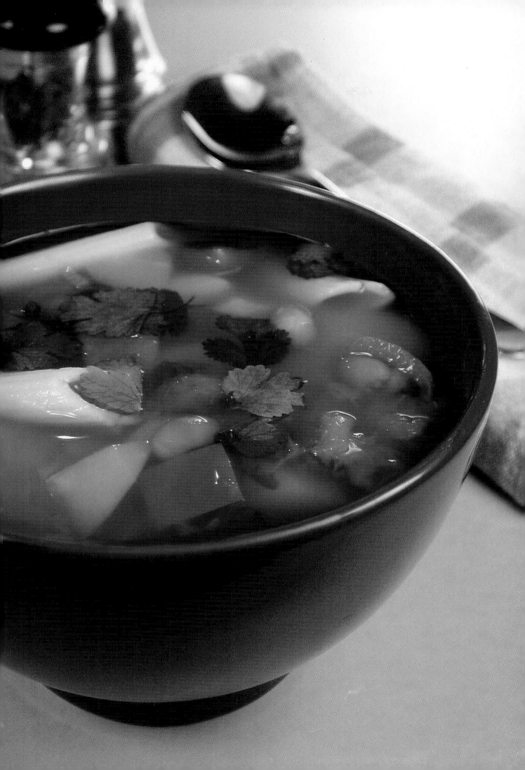

Corn Soup with Ginger, Chilli & Coriander

(pictured on front cover, top left)

1 onion, chopped
1 carrot, very thinly sliced
1 zucchini, very thinly sliced
2 tspns chicken stock powder
1 tbspn fresh grated ginger
1/2 tspn minced garlic
2 tspns chilli paste
1 tspn ground coriander
4 1/2 cups water
1 x 400g can chickpeas, rinsed and drained (optional)
1 x 420g can creamed corn
3 tbspns chopped coriander leaves
fish sauce to taste

Combine onion, carrot, zucchini, chicken stock powder, ginger, garlic, chilli paste, ground coriander and 1/2 cup water in a large saucepan. Cook 5 minutes.
Add remaining water, chickpeas and creamed corn and bring to boil, then lower heat, cover and simmer for 10 minutes. Stir occasionally. Stir through the coriander leaves and add fish sauce to taste, and serve. Serves 4.

♥ approx. 2g fat per serve

Lite Laksa

Here is my lite version of a traditionally very high fat dish. Coconut milk, the main ingredient in Laksa is very high in fat, and the fat is mostly saturated fat. A traditional Laksa can contain up to 40g fat in one serve!

1 x 125g chicken breast fillet, skinned and all visible fat removed,
3/4 cup evaporated low-fat milk
1 tspn coconut essence
1 heaped tspn cornflour
2 cakes rice noodles (fat-free)
1/2 jar John West Singapore Laksa Paste
1 1/4 cups water
1 tspn sugar
2 green chillies, chopped (optional)
6 mushrooms, quartered
2 small carrots, sliced
2 spring onions, sliced into 3 cm slices
4 snow peas, sliced
garnish:
cucumber slices
bean shoots
fresh mint
fresh coriander

Cook the chicken (steam or microwave) and cut into 1 cm dice.
Combine evaporated skim milk, coconut essence and cornflour thoroughly and set aside.
Cook rice noodles according to packet directions, and drain.
In a saucepan, simmer Laksa Paste, water, sugar and chillies for 2 minutes. Add milk mixture to saucepan and simmer 2 minutes, stirring constantly to prevent catching on bottom. Add mushrooms, carrots, spring onions and snow peas. Simmer 2 minutes.
Prepare 2 bowls by placing noodles and chicken in base. Pour soup over top and garnish with cucumber, bean shoots, mint and coriander.
Serves 2.

♥ approx. 4·5g fat per serve

Curried Pumpkin, Apple & Ginger Soup

1 tspn ground coriander
1 tspn grated ginger
1 tbspn Indian curry powder
600g chopped pumpkin
1 large onion, chopped
1 granny smith apple, peeled, cored and chopped
1 litre fat-free chicken stock

Cook coriander, ginger and curry powder in a little of the stock.
Add pumpkin, onion, apple and a little more stock.
Cover and cook over very low heat 15 minutes, adding extra stock as necessary to prevent sticking to base.
Blend soup with 2 cups of stock. Return to pan. Add remaining stock and reheat.
Season with salt and freshly ground black pepper. Serves 4.

♥ under ·5g per serve

Spiced Bean, Pasta & Tomato Soup

2 carrots, chopped
1 onion, finely chopped
2 1/2 cups fat-free vegetable stock
1 green capsicum, chopped
2 x 800g cans tomatoes with their juice
1 x 420g can kidney beans, rinsed and drained
1 tbspn hot curry powder
1 tspn ground cardamom
1 tspn ground cinnamon
1/4 tspn ground cloves
2 cups cooked pasta spirals
1/2 cup coriander leaves

Place carrot, onion and stock in a stockpot and cook covered for 5 minutes.
Add capsicum, tomatoes and beans and continue cooking. Meanwhile, combine spices in a non-stick pan and heat until aromatic. Toss them around so you do not burn them.
Add spices to stockpot and bring soup to the boil. Lower heat and simmer uncovered 5 minutes.
Add pasta and cook 2-3 minutes. Stir in coriander. Serves 6.

♥ approx. ·5g fat per serve

Spiced Zucchini Soup with Rice Noodle Salad

1 onion, sliced
1 large leek, (white part only) sliced
1 small red chilli finely chopped
1/2 tspn minced ginger
1/2 tspn minced garlic
2 Kaffir lime leaves*
1 stick lemon grass, cut in half and bruised
2 tbspns chopped fresh coriander leaves
2 1/2 cups hot fat-free vegetable stock
4 zucchinis, chopped
200mls evaporated low-fat milk
1 tspn coconut essence
1/2 tspn cornflour
2 tbspns fish sauce
1 tbspn lime juice

Noodle Salad:
150g rice noodles, (dry weight) cooked and drained
1/2 red onion, sliced finely
1/2 red capsicum, sliced finely
1/4 cup fresh coriander leaves
2 tspns chopped fresh mint leaves
1 tbspn lime juice
1 tbspn Char Sui sauce (available from supermarket)

In a large pot, cook the first eight ingredients over medium heat in a little of the stock, 4-5 minutes. Add extra stock if needed. Add zucchini and cook 5 minutes or until onion is transparent.
Combine milk with cornflour and essence and then add to pot with all the remaining soup ingredients. Bring to the boil and simmer 15-20 minutes or until the zucchini is soft.
Meanwhile combine all the noodle salad ingredients and toss to coat with the sauce.
Remove lemongrass and lime leaves from the soup and puree the mixture. Serve in bowls topped with noodle salad. Serves 4 generously.

♥ approx. ·8g fat per serve

Pumpkin & Basil Soup

1 kg chopped butternut pumpkin
2 leeks, chopped
2 heaped tspns dried basil leaves
6 cups water
3 tspns vegetable stock powder
3 tbspns tomato paste
1 tbspn minced ginger
2 tspns minced garlic
2 tbspns sweet chilli sauce
freshly ground black pepper to taste
1 tbspn orange juice

Combine all the ingredients except orange juice in a stockpot and bring
to the boil. Lower heat and simmer, covered for 10 minutes.
Remove cover and simmer further 5-8 minutes or until pumpkin is very
soft. Add orange juice and puree the soup. Serves 4.

♥ neg. fat per serve

Mushroom Soup (Microwave)

1/2 cup evaporated low-fat milk
1 tspn cornflour
250g mushrooms, sliced
1 tbspn balsamic vinegar
2 cups fat-free chicken stock
1/4 cup white wine
1 tspn French mustard
1 tbspn fresh chopped chives
plain non-fat yoghurt to serve
freshly ground black pepper to taste

Combine evaporated milk and cornflour thoroughly.
Place mushrooms and balsamic vinegar in a microwave-proof dish,
cover and cook 4 minutes HIGH.
Add chicken stock, wine, mustard and milk mixture, cover and cook 10
minutes HIGH.
Puree soup and serve with chives, yoghurt and pepper. Serves 4.

♥ approx. ·75g fat per serve

Lentil & Sweet Potato Soup

1 small brown onion, finely chopped
1/2 tspn minced garlic
2 tspns ground cumin
1 tspn ground coriander
1/4 tspn chilli powder
1/4 tspn turmeric
1/2 tspn ground cinnamon
1 cup red lentils, rinsed and drained
1 kg sweet potato, peeled and chopped into 2cm pieces
5 cups fat-free vegetable stock
freshly ground black pepper and sea salt to taste
1/4 cup chopped fresh coriander leaves

Place onion, garlic, cumin, coriander, chilli powder, turmeric and
cinnamon in a large saucepan with a little stock and cook until it is
aromatic.
Add lentils, sweet potato and stock. Bring to the boil, then reduce heat
to medium low and simmer covered for 10 minutes, stirring frequently.
Remove lid and cook uncovered for a further 10 minutes or until sweet
potato and lentils are soft enough to mash. Mash the mixture with a
potato masher.
Add salt and pepper to taste.
Remove from heat and stir through coriander leaves. Serve with fresh hot
bread. Serves 4.

♥ approx. 1g fat per serve

Tomato Corn Soup

1 onion, chopped
1 tspn chicken stock powder
1 tspn ground coriander
1 x 400g tin tomatoes, chopped with the juice
1 1/2 cups tomato puree
2 tspns dried parsley
1 x 420g tin creamed corn
1 x 420g tin corn kernels
1/4 tspn chilli powder
chopped fresh mint to serve

Cook onion, stock powder and coriander in a little tomato juice from the can, until onion is soft. Add remaining ingredients, except mint and cook until heated through. Serve with mint. Serves 4.

♥ approx. 1·5g fat per serve

Creamy Corn & Tarragon Soup

1 large potato, chopped
1 large onion, chopped
4 cups skim milk
1 bay leaf
1 x 400g can corn kernels
1 tbspn cornflour combined with 3 tbspns water
1 red capsicum, chopped
1 x 420g can creamed corn
2 tbspns chopped parsley
2 tbspns tarragon mustard
2-3 tbspns sweet chilli sauce
1 diced tomato
salt and pepper to taste

Combine potato, onion, milk and bay leaf in a large saucepan with half of the sweet corn kernels.
Bring to boil, then cover and simmer on low heat until potato is soft, approximately 15 minutes. Stir occasionally to ensure milk does not catch on base of pan.
Remove bay leaf and then puree mixture. Return to pan and add cornflour mixture and stir through.
Add remaining ingredients and return to heat. Stir until heated through and soup has thickened. Serves 4.

♥ approx. 1·6g fat per serve

Living Lite

pasta

Photo right: *Linguine with Eggplant, Chickpeas, Coriander & Mint (recipe page 28)*

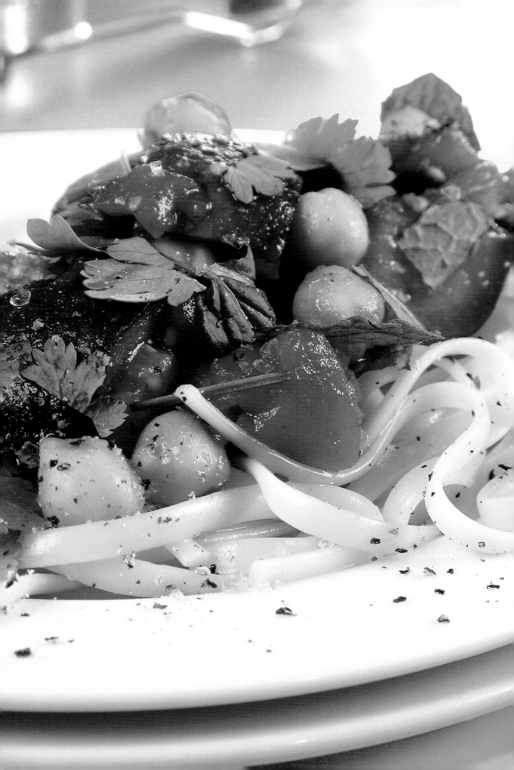

Penne with Tuna, Chilli & Coriander Sauce

non-stick oil spray
1 onion, chopped
1 tspn minced garlic
1/2 tspn ground coriander
1 x 800g tin chopped tomatoes
2 cups chopped broccoli
1 tspn lemongrass
1 tspn chilli flakes
1 x 425g can tuna in spring water, drained and flaked (John West)
1/2 cup chopped fresh coriander
freshly ground black pepper to taste
250g penne, cooked to serve

Spray a non-stick pan very lightly with oil spray. Add onion, garlic and ground coriander. Cook 1 minute, then add a little water to prevent sticking. Cook until onion is soft.
Add tomatoes, broccoli, lemon grass, chilli and tuna. Cook 10 minutes, stirring occasionally. Add the coriander and pepper to taste and serve over penne. Serves 4.

♥ approx. 1·5g fat per serve

Linguine with Eggplant, Chickpeas, Coriander & Mint

oil-water spray (page 131)
1 eggplant, washed
1/2 tspn minced garlic
Balsamic vinegar
1 x 400g can chopped tomatoes
1/2 tspn ground cinnamon
1 cup drained canned chickpeas
2 tbspns sweet chilli sauce
2 tbspns chopped fresh coriander leaves
1 tbspn chopped fresh mint
good pinch sea salt
freshly ground black pepper to taste
cooked linguine to serve

Prick eggplant all over with a fork, and microwave 2-3 minutes HIGH.
Place in a plastic bag and leave few minutes. Cut eggplant into cubes.
Place garlic in a wok and spray with oil-water spray. Add 1 tbspn of
balsamic vinegar and the tomatoes. Cook on low heat for 5 minutes.
Add cinnamon, chickpeas, another 1 tbspn balsamic vinegar, eggplant
cubes and chilli sauce and cook gently until sauce is hot. Stir through
coriander and mint.
Check for seasoning, adding pepper and salt to taste. Serve over linguine.
Serves 4.

♥approx. ·5g fat per serve

Pasta with Ricotta, Broccoli & Mushrooms

1 large onion, chopped
2 large ripe tomatoes, chopped
1 cup sliced mushrooms
2 cups chopped broccoli or spinach leaves
1/2 cup low-fat ricotta cheese
freshly ground black pepper to taste
400g penne pasta, cooked and kept warm

Cook onion and tomatoes in a pan (or microwave) until the tomatoes are very soft.
Add mushrooms and broccoli or spinach and cook until tender or the spinach wilts.
Mix ricotta through hot mixture to form a sauce. Stir through pasta. Add pepper to taste. Serves 4.

♥ approx. 2·5g fat per serve

Chicken & Asparagus Pasta Sauce (Microwave)

1 spring onion, sliced
1 tspn white mustard seeds
1 tbspn hot chilli sauce
1/2 cup fat-free vegetable stock
150g cooked chicken breast cubes
2 tbspns chopped capers
1 bunch fresh asparagus, sliced into 4
1 red capsicum, chopped
1 tspn pine nuts (optional)
300ml skim milk combined with 1 tspn cornflour
1 tspn dried dill
1/4 tspn white pepper
1 tbspn fresh basil
2 tbspns lemon juice
400g pasta of your choice, cooked and kept warm

Place the spring onion, mustard seeds and chilli sauce in a wok, with 1 tbspn stock. Cook over medium to high heat 1 minute.
Add chicken pieces, capers and asparagus. Stir 1 minute, adding extra stock as necessary. Add capsicum, pine nuts and cook 1 minute. Add milk and cook over medium heat. Add remaining ingredients and stir until mixture thickens.
Serve tossed through hot pasta. Serves 4.

♥ approx. 1·5g fat per serve (without pine nuts)
♥ approx. 3·7g fat per serve (with pine nuts)

Risoni with Chicken, Zucchini & Mushrooms

oil-water spray (page 131)
2 cups sliced mushrooms
1 cup chopped onion
2 tspns minced garlic
1 tbspn chicken seasoning (eg. Masterfoods)
3 tspns chicken stock powder
salt & freshly ground black pepper to taste
1 3/4 cups risoni*
4 cups boiling water
2 cups sliced zucchini
1/2 cup chopped red capsicum
250g diced chicken breast fillets (skinned and all visible fat
removed) cooked
1 cup thawed frozen peas
2 tbspns chopped fresh parsley
2 tbspns low-fat ricotta cheese

Spray a large stockpot with oil-water spray and add mushrooms, onion, garlic, chicken seasoning and stock powder and salt and pepper. Cook 3-4 minutes.
Add risoni and 1/2 cup boiling water. Cook until risoni absorbs all the water. Gradually add remaining water, stirring the whole time until all the water has been added. Cook 5 minutes, add zucchini and capsicum and cook 5 minutes more or until risoni is 'al dente'.
Add the cooked chicken, peas, parsley and ricotta cheese and stir until heated through. Serves 6.

♥ approx. 2·5g fat per serve

Spaghetti With Asian Herbs

(pictured on front cover, bottom left)

1 x 500g packet thin spaghetti
1/2 cup sliced mushrooms
1 cup chopped broccoli
5 stalks asparagus, quartered
1/4 cup chopped red capsicum
1 cup chopped fresh basil leaves
1/2 cup chopped fresh mint
1/2 cup chopped fresh coriander
1 tspn chilli paste
1 tbspn sweet chilli sauce
2/3 cup low-salt soy sauce
1 tbspn sugar or Splenda
2 tbspns lime juice
1/3 cup mirin*

Cook pasta according to directions.
Steam or microwave mushrooms, broccoli, asparagus and capsicum.
Drain well and then add to the pasta with the basil, mint and coriander.
Stir through.
Combine chilli paste, chilli sauce, soy sauce, sugar or Splenda, lime
juice and mirin.
Pour over pasta and stir through until pasta is coated in the sauce. Serve
immediately. Serves 4.

♥ approx. 2g fat per serve

Fettucine With Pumpkin, Lemon & Spinach

375g fettucine, dry weight
1 onion, chopped
1/2 tspn minced garlic
600g butternut pumpkin, peeled and chopped into 2 cm pieces
1 tspn chopped fresh rosemary leaves
juice 1 lemon
1 tspn lemon rind
1 x 250g packet frozen spinach, thawed and drained
1 cup plain non-fat yoghurt
1/3 cup no-oil French dressing
1 tspn cornflour
salt and freshly ground black pepper to taste

Cook fettucine, drain, set aside and keep warm.
Cook onion and garlic in 1 tbspn water until the onion is soft (or microwave 3 minutes HIGH).
Add pumpkin, rosemary and 1/4 cup water. Cook covered until pumpkin is soft and most of the water has evaporated (or microwave 8 minutes HIGH covered and 2 minutes uncovered).
Add lemon juice, rind and spinach.
Combine yoghurt, dressing and cornflour and toss through pasta. Toss pumpkin mixture through pasta.
Reheat gently. Add salt and freshly ground black pepper to taste.
Serves 4.

♥ approx. 1·5g fat per serve

Spinach, Rocket & Mushroom Pasta Sauce

1 x 250g packet frozen spinach, thawed
small bunch rocket leaves, roughly chopped
5 large mushrooms, sliced
1 tbspn lemon juice
1 tbspn white wine vinegar
3-4 spring onions, sliced
freshly ground black pepper
1/2 cup Slimmer Sour Cream (page 132)
1/2 cup tomato puree
1/2 tspn cornflour
1 tbspn hot chilli sauce
hot cooked pasta to serve

Cook spinach, rocket, mushrooms and lemon juice in the wine vinegar for 2 minutes. Combine remaining ingredients together thoroughly and add to the pan. Toss through hot cooked pasta. Serves 4.

♥ approx. 2g fat per serve (sauce only)

Creamy Tomato & Vegetable Sauce

1 red capsicum, cut into large flat pieces
1 x 340g block silken tofu, drained
3 tbspns tomato paste
1 cup fat-free vegetable stock
1 tbspn white wine vinegar
2 tspns Spicy Italian seasoning
1 small brown onion, chopped
1 tspn minced garlic
2 bunches asparagus, trimmed and sliced
100g sliced mushrooms
1 x 400g tin chopped tomatoes
chilli flakes to taste
1/4 cup fresh parsley leaves, chopped
freshly ground black pepper
400g pasta of your choice, cooked and kept warm

Roast capsicum by placing pieces under a hot grill and cooking until the skin blackens and chars. Place the pieces into a plastic bag to cool and then peel off the skin when cooled slightly.
Puree tofu, tomato paste, vegetable stock, vinegar, and seasoning until smooth.
In a saucepan, cook onion, garlic and asparagus with a little water 3-5 minutes and add then mushrooms and capsicums. Cook further 3-5 minutes and then add pureed mixture.
Add tomatoes, chilli, parsley and pepper and cook 5 minutes. Serve over hot pasta. Serves 4.

♥ approx. 1g fat per serve

Creamy Spiced Vegetable Pasta Sauce

Balsamic vinegar
1 onion, chopped
1/4 red capsicum, chopped
1 carrot, diced
2 cups chopped broccoli
2 cups sliced mushrooms
8 sun-dried tomatoes, (not in oil), chopped
3/4 cup plain non-fat yoghurt
1/4 cup skim milk
1 heaped tbspn cornflour
1/4 cup chopped fresh parsley
1 tspn dried dill
good pinch nutmeg
good pinch cinnamon
2 tspns sweet chilli sauce
freshly ground black pepper
hot pasta to serve

Add 1 tbspn balsamic vinegar to a non-stick pan. Add onion, and capsicum and cook until onion is soft.
Add carrot, cook 1 minute and add broccoli, mushrooms and sun-dried tomatoes. Add extra balsamic vinegar as needed to prevent vegetables from sticking.
In a bowl or jug, combine remaining ingredients together. Add to pan and stir until sauce thickens slightly. Toss through hot pasta. Serves 4.

♥ less than ·5g fat per serve (sauce only)

Living Lite

chicken

Photo right: *Chicken & Onion in Sweet Chilli & Ginger Sauce*
(recipe page 41)

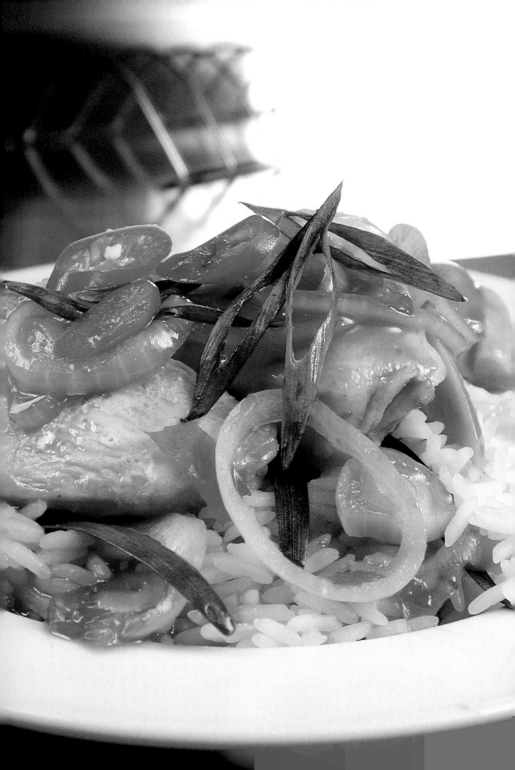

Apricot Mango & Mint Chicken

1 x 825g tin apricots, drained, liquid reserved
1 tbspn hot mango chutney
freshly ground black pepper
1/4 tspn dried sage
1/4 tspn ground cinnamon
1 tspn grated ginger
1/2 tspn minced garlic
1 tbspn lemon juice
4 x 125g chicken breast fillets, skinned and all visible fat removed
1 tbspn dried onion flakes
1 1/2 tbspns cornflour combined with 2 tbspns water
1 tbspn chopped fresh mint leaves

Preheat oven to 180°C.
Puree apricots, mango chutney, pepper, sage, cinnamon, ginger garlic and lemon juice.
Place chicken in a shallow casserole dish in a single layer. Season with extra pepper and sprinkle onion flakes over top of chicken.
Pour pureed apricot over chicken evenly. Bake 30 minutes.
Remove from oven, remove chicken pieces and set aside in a dish and cover with foil to keep warm.
Pour reserved liquid into a small saucepan and add cornflour paste.
Heat, stirring constantly until the sauce thickens.
Place chicken into a clean serving platter and pour sauce over. Sprinkle with mint. Serve with rice and a salad. Serves 4.

♥ approx. 1·5g fat per serve

Creamy Mushroom & Chive
Chicken Casserole

1 x 150g chicken breast fillet, skinned and all visible fat removed
2 single serve packets diet mushroom and chive soup mix
1/2 cup evaporated low-fat milk
6 mushrooms, sliced
1 spring onion, finely sliced
1 small onion, sliced into rings
1 tbspn red wine
dash Worcestershire sauce
pinch cayenne pepper
1/2 cup plain non-fat yoghurt, combined with 1 tbspn cornflour

Cook the chicken (steam or microwave) and cut into 1 cm dice.
Combine the soup mixes with the milk in a small jug, using a whisk.
Cook (or microwave 4 minutes on high) mushrooms, spring onion and
onion until soft.
Add wine, soup mixture, Worcestershire sauce and cayenne pepper.
Cook (or microwave further 2 minutes).
Add chicken and yoghurt mixture and heat gently until chicken is
heated through. Serve with rice or toast. Serves 2.

♥ approx. 3g fat per serve

Chicken & Onion in Sweet Chilli & Ginger Sauce (Microwave)

500g chicken breast, skinned and all visible fat removed
1 onion, sliced
1 tspn ginger
1/2 tspn minced garlic
1/4 tspn dried chilli flakes
1 tbspn hoi sin sauce
1 tbspn sweet chilli sauce
1 tbspn oyster sauce
3 drops sesame oil (optional)

Slice chicken into 1·5 cm slices, and steam or microwave until just cooked.
Place onion, ginger, garlic and chilli flakes in a microwave-proof casserole dish with 1 tbspn water. Cover and microwave for 2 minutes on HIGH.
Stir and add remaining ingredients and chicken.
Cover and microwave 4 minutes on HIGH. Serve with rice. Serves 2.

♥ approx. 2·5g fat per serve

Chicken With Nuts & Sultanas (Microwave)

500g chicken breast, skinned and all visible fat removed
2 tbspns sultanas
1 tbspn peanuts, chopped
1 tbspn cashews, chopped
1 tbspn Chinese cooking wine
100mls fat-free chicken stock
1 tspn cinnamon
2 tbspn chopped parsley
freshly ground black pepper
1 heaped tspn cornflour

Slice chicken into large slices (approx 5cm x 3cm).
Place sultanas, nuts, cooking wine and stock in a microwave-proof
casserole dish, Cover and microwave 2 minutes HIGH.
Add chicken and all remaining ingredients except cornflour and
microwave covered 6-8 minutes, stirring halfway through cooking.
Combine cornflour with a little water to form a paste and stir thoroughly
through chicken.
Microwave 1-2 minutes until sauce thickens. Serve with rice. Serves 4.

♥ approx. 5g fat per serve

Mustard Baked Chicken

1/2 cup oil-free Italian dressing
1/4 cup soy sauce
1/4 cup finely chopped spring onions
1 tspn dry mustard powder
freshly ground black pepper
4 x 125g chicken breast fillets, skinned and all visible fat removed

Preheat oven to 200°C.
Combine dressing, soy sauce, onion and mustard.
Place chicken in an ovenproof casserole dish. Pour dressing mixture over chicken. Sprinkle with pepper.
Cover dish with foil. Bake 40 to 45 minutes, then remove foil and bake until chicken is a golden brown. Serves 4.

♥ approx. 1·5g fat per serve

Honey Mustard Crumbed Chicken

4 x 125g chicken breast fillets, skinned and all visible fat removed
1/4 cup German mustard
1/4 cup honey
1/2 tspn minced garlic
salt and freshly ground black pepper
cornflake crumbs

Preheat oven to 180°C.
Combine mustard, honey, garlic salt and pepper in a bowl.
Coat each chicken fillets in the mixture, then roll in cornflake crumbs.
Place fillets on a non-stick oven tray lined with baking paper and bake
30-35 minutes. Serves 4.

♥ approx. 1·5g fat per serve

Coriander Cardamom Chicken

2 tspns ground coriander
1 tspn ground cardamom
1/2 tspn grated ginger
1/2 tspn ground cloves
1 tspn black pepper
1/2 tspn salt
1 cup plain non-fat yoghurt
4 x 125g chicken breast fillets, skinned and all visible fat removed

Preheat oven to 180°C.
Combine all ingredients except chicken. Coat chicken in marinade and refrigerate at least two hours.
Place fillets on a non-stick oven tray lined with baking paper and bake 30-35 minutes or grill on a barbecue plate. Serves 4.

♥ approx. 1·5g fat per serve

Green Thai Chicken Curry

500g chicken breast fillets, skinned and all visible fat removed
2 x 375 ml cans evaporated low-fat milk
3 tspns coconut essence
2 tspns cornflour
1 tbspn fat-free Thai curry paste*
1 tbspn sliced lemongrass
3 green chillies, finely chopped
1 bunch coriander, roughly chopped
1 tbspn fish sauce
lime juice to taste
1/2 cup torn basil leaves

Cut chicken into strips and set aside.
Thoroughly combine evaporated milk, coconut essence and cornflour in a jug and set aside.
Dry fry curry paste in a non-stick wok or pan, adding a little water if necessary.
Add lemongrass and evaporated milk mixture to pan. Stir until the mixture thickens slightly.
Add chicken and chillies and simmer on low heat until chicken is cooked through. Remove from heat and add coriander.
Season to taste with the fish sauce and lime juice.
Stir through basil leaves just before serving with rice. Serves 4.

♥ approx. 3g fat per serve

Chicken In Lime, Mint & Coriander Marinade

500g chicken breast fillets, skinned and all visible fat removed
1 1/2 cups plain non-fat yoghurt
8 finely shredded kaffir lime leaves*
2 tbspns finely chopped mint leaves
2 tbspns finely chopped coriander leaves
1/2 tspn ground cumin
1/2 tspn ground coriander
1/2 cup lime juice
1 lime, cut into wedges, to serve

Wash the chicken fillets and pat dry with paper towel. Cut a few shallow cuts into each fillet.
Combine remaining ingredients and add chicken. Turn to coat with marinade and refrigerate at least 2 hours.
Preheat oven to 180°C.
Bake chicken fillets on a non-stick oven tray 35-40 minutes.
Garnish with extra coriander leaves and lime wedges. Serves 4.

♥ approx. 1·5g fat per serve

Chicken with Curry & Marmalade Sauce

500g chicken breast fillets, skinned and all visible fat removed
1 tbspn soy sauce
1 1/2 tbspns fat-free curry paste*
1/2 tspn minced garlic
1/2 cup sugar-free orange marmalade (eg.Monbulk)
1 1/2 tbspns lime juice
3/4 cup plain non-fat yoghurt

Wash the chicken fillets and pat dry with paper towel. Cut into stir-fry strips.
Cook chicken strips in soy sauce over low heat until browned.
Remove chicken from pan and wipe out pan.
Add curry paste, garlic, marmalade and lime juice to the pan and cook 1 minute. Remove pan from heat and stir yoghurt through thoroughly.
Add chicken to pan and toss to coat in sauce. Serve immediately.
Serves 4.

♥ approx. 1·5g fat per serve

Living Lite

fish & seafood

Photo right: *Thai Style Fishcakes with Yoghurt & Mint Sauce*
(recipe page 58)

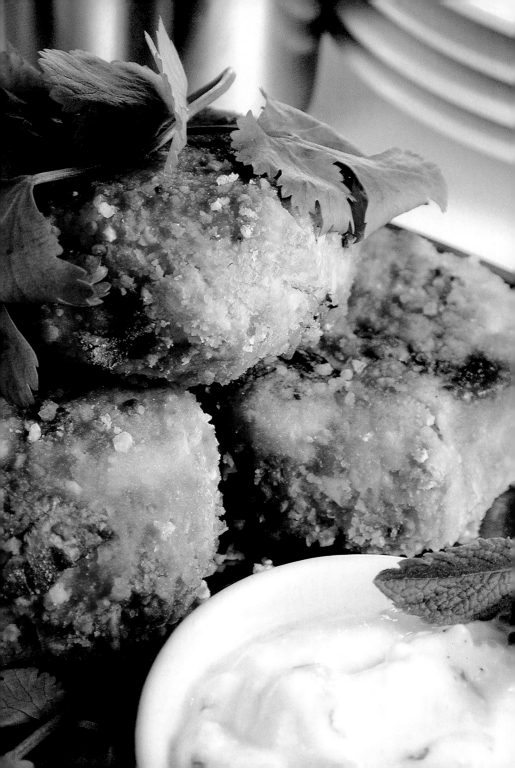

Lemon Pepper Fish with Dill Mustard Dressing

2 x 150g fish fillets (eg. bream, John Dory)
lemon pepper seasoning (Masterfood's)

dressing:
1/2 cup plain non-fat yoghurt
1/4 tspn dried dill
1 tspn Dijon mustard
1/8 tspn lemon juice
1 tbspn chopped dried apple
white pepper

Combine dressing ingredients and set aside.
Sprinkle lemon pepper over fish and rub into surface.
Grill on a hot barbecue plate or similar, until cooked approximately 2-3 minutes each side. Do not overcook.
Serve fish with dressing drizzled over top. Serves 2.

♥ approx. 2g fat per serve

Tuna & Corn Mix

1 small onion, chopped
1/2 cup chopped dried apple
1 heaped tspn dried dill
4 heaped tbspns Dijon mustard
1 green capsicum, chopped
1 x 425g can tuna in springwater, drained and flaked (John West)
1 small can corn kernels
1 x 420g can creamed corn
white pepper to taste
1 tspn lemon juice

Cook onion in a little water until soft.
Add dried apple and extra 1/4 cup water. Cook further 5 minutes. Add dill, mustard and capsicum. Cook 5 minutes.
Add tuna, corn kernels, creamed corn, pepper and lemon juice and heat through.
Serve with couscous, rice, pasta or potatoes. Serves 4.

♥ less than 2g fat per serve

Tuna & White Bean Loaf

1 x 425g tin tuna in springwater, drained and flaked (John West)
1/2 cup canned white beans, drained, rinsed and dried
1 cup rolled oats
2 egg whites or substitute*
1 cup grated carrot
1 cup chopped mushrooms
1 tbspn chopped fresh dill
1/2 cup chopped spring onions
1/2 tspn sea salt
1 1/2 tbspns Dijon mustard
1 tbspn currants

Preheat oven to 180°C.
Line a large non-stick loaf tin with baking paper.
Combine all ingredients and place in loaf tin. Bake 45 minutes.
Stand 5 minutes before removing from tin and slicing. Serves 4.

♥ approx. 3·5g fat per serve

Crumbed Crab Cakes

4 cups crab meat (fresh or canned)
2 tbspns lemon juice
1 spring onion, chopped
1/3 cup red capsicum, finely chopped.
2 cups fresh breadcrumbs (made from 3-4 slices fat-free bread)
1/4 cup fat-free mayonnaise (page 132) or 98% fat-free mayonnaise
(Kraft or Freedom Foods)
2 egg whites or substitute, lightly beaten
1 tspn seafood seasoning
freshly ground black pepper to taste
1/2 tspn Tabasco sauce
1/2 cup cornflake crumbs

Preheat oven to 200°C. Line a non-stick oven tray with baking paper.
Combine crabmeat with all the ingredients except cornflake crumbs, in
a large bowl. Stir together well and form 6 thick patties. Roll in dry
cornflake crumbs.
Cook patties on a non-stick pan over medium heat until golden, only 1
minute each side. Carefully, turn over and transfer to the oven tray.
Bake 10-12 minutes, or until heated through.
Serve with seafood sauce (page 137)

♥ approx. 2·5g fat per serve (with commercial mayonnaise)

Salmon And Asparagus with Pasta in Dill & Lime Sauce

1 x 175g salmon fillet
2 1/2 tbspns lime juice
verjuice*
freshly ground black pepper
1/2 cup fat-free vegetable stock
6 Kaffir lime leaves*, finely sliced
1 tbspn chopped capers
1 tbspn Dijon mustard
2 tspns dried dill
1/2 tspn wasabi powder*
1 bunch fresh asparagus, trimmed and quartered
1 cup skim milk combined with 1 tspn cornflour
hot pasta to serve

Combine 2 tspns lime juice, 2 tbspns verjuice and some freshly ground black pepper in a frypan. Add the salmon fillet and cook 2-3 minutes each side or until just cooked. Remove from the pan and set aside to cool.
Swirl 1 tspn verjuice in pan and using a wooden or plastic spatula, work off any of the juices and remainder of the salmon from the bottom of the pan. Pour this over the salmon fillet.
In a small saucepan, place the stock, remaining lime juice, lime leaves, capers, mustard, dill, wasabi powder and asparagus and cook 2-3 minutes over medium heat. Lower the heat, add milk, and cook further 2 minutes, stirring.
Slice the salmon fillet thickly and add with the juices to the sauce and reheat. Serve over hot pasta. Serves 4.

♥ approx. 2·75g fat per serve (without pasta)

Tuna Fish Cakes with Lemongrass, Lime & Ginger

2 x 185g cans tuna with lemongrass, lime and ginger in spring-water
(John West brand)
1/4 cup finely chopped spring onions
4 egg whites or substitute, lightly beaten
2 tbspns lime juice
freshly ground black pepper to taste
1/2 cup crushed low-fat crispbread crumbs (eg. 98% fat-free Salada
biscuits)
1 cup cornflake crumbs

Drain and flake the tuna and place in a large bowl with all the
ingredients except cornflake crumbs.
Mix well and shape into 8 patties. Roll patties in the cornflake crumbs
to coat.
Spray a non-stick pan very lightly with non-stick vegetable oil spray.
Cook patties 5-6 minutes each side or until brown. Serves 6.

♥ under ·5g fat per patty

Grilled Fish in Chilli, Lime & Lemongrass Marinade

4 x 150g thick white firm fish fillets (eg cod)

marinade:
1/2 cup chopped spring onions
1 tspn minced garlic
2 tbspns lime juice
1-2 tspns hot chilli paste (fat-free)
2 tbspns teriyaki sauce
2 tbspns fish sauce
1 tspn honey
1 tbspn finely chopped lemongrass

Combine the marinade ingredients in a large baking dish.
Place the fish in marinade and turn to coat. Cover and refrigerate for at least one hour.
Line a griller plate with alfoil and spray very lightly with non-stick vegetable spray.
Cook the fillets on griller plate 4 minutes each side.
Serve immediately. Serves 4.

♥ under 1g fat per serve

Thai Style Fish Cakes with Yoghurt & Mint Sauce

2 cups cooked plain mashed potatoes
1 x 425g can tuna in spring-water, drained and flaked (John West)
1 small onion, finely chopped
1/4 cup fresh coriander, chopped
1 tbspn fresh grated ginger
2 small chillies, finely chopped
2 egg whites or substitute*
salt and freshly ground black pepper to taste
1 cup dry breadcrumbs
soy sauce

Yoghurt & Mint Sauce:
1 cup plain non-fat yoghurt
3 spring onions, finely sliced
3 tspns chopped fresh mint
salt & pepper

In a large bowl combine the tuna and mashed potatoes.
Add onion, coriander, ginger, chilli, egg whites, salt and pepper. Mix
well and shape into 8 patties. Coat each patty with the breadcrumbs.
Using a pastry brush, "paint" each patty with a little soy sauce.
Lightly spray a non-stick pan with a little vegetable oil and cook patties
on both sides.
Combine all the sauce ingredients thoroughly.
Serve the fishcakes with the sauce.

♥ approx. ·5g fat per fish cake

Fish Baked in a Parcel with Chilli, Mint & Coriander

4 x 150g thick white firm fish fillets (eg cod)
1/2 cup chopped spring onions
1/3 cup plain non-fat yoghurt
1 tbspn chopped fresh mint
1 tbspn chopped fresh coriander
2 tbspns sweet chilli sauce

Preheat oven to 180°C.
Place each fish fillet on a piece of alfoil large enough to wrap around the fish to form a sealed parcel.
Combine yoghurt with remaining ingredients and spread over each fillet.
Fold alfoil into a parcel sealing edges completely.
Bake 15-20 minutes. Serves 4.

♥ approx. 1g fat per serve

Tuscan Spiced Crumbed Fish

4 x 150g firm white fish fillets (eg cod)
1/2 cup plain non-fat yoghurt
1 1/2 tspns balsamic vinegar
1/2 tspn dijon mustard
1 cup dry breadcrumbs
2 tbspns Tuscan seasoning (Masterfoods brand)

Line a griller plate with alfoil and spray very lightly with non-stick vegetable spray.
Wash and pat dry fish fillets.
Combine yoghurt, vinegar and mustard in a wide bowl.
Combine breadcrumbs with Tuscan seasoning and spread out on a plate.
Coat fish in yoghurt mixture, then roll in combined breadcrumb mixture.
Place fillets on grill plate and grill 4 minutes each side. Serve immediately. Serves 4.

♥ approx. 1·5g fat per serve

Living Lite

vegetarian mains

Photo right: *Pumpkin, Spinach & Cottage Cheese Tart*
(recipe page 67)

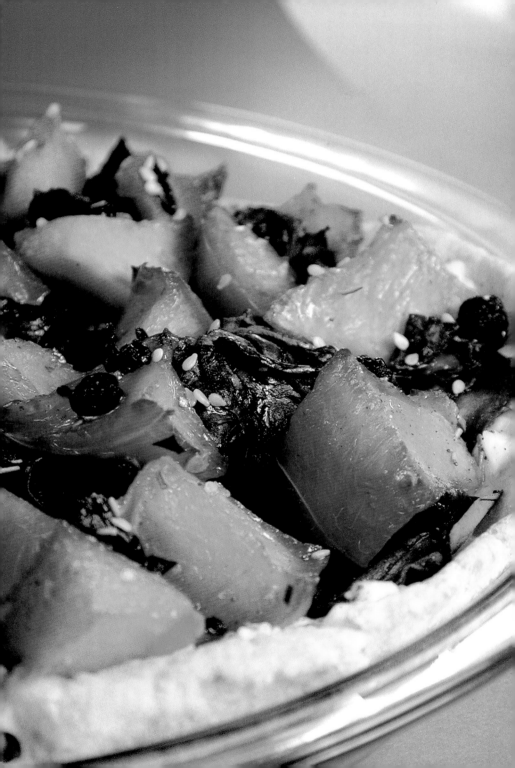

Easy Spinach & Mushroom Risotto

3 spring onions, chopped
1 leek sliced
1 tspn minced garlic
1/2 cup white wine
2 cups arborio rice
1 x 250g packet frozen spinach, thawed and drained
8 sun dried tomatoes, soaked and chopped
6 mushrooms, sliced
1/2 tspn salt
1/4 tspn saffron powder
1/2 tspn dried chives
1/2 tspn dried thyme
1 tbspns dried parsley
6 cups good strong fat-free vegetable stock
freshly round black pepper to taste

"Saute" spring onions, leek and garlic in a little of the wine, until the onion is transparent.
Add rice and vegetables and stir through.
Add remaining wine, herbs, salt and saffron powder.
Add stock and stir well. Bring to boil, then lower heat and cook slowly, stirring occasionally 15-20 minutes.
Season with black pepper. Serves 4-6.

♥ for 4 approx. ·5g fat per serve
♥ for 6 approx. ·3g fat per serve

Thai Rice (Microwave)

1 medium onion, chopped
1/2 tspn minced garlic
1 tbspn lime juice
1 tspn ground coriander
good pinch cardamom powder
3 cups water
1 1/2 tspns chicken stock powder
1 1/3 cups jasmine rice
1 tspn chilli paste (or more to taste)
1/4 tspn lemon grass powder
2 dried kaffir lime leaves*, crumbled
1 x 400g tin crushed pineapple, drained
2 tbspns chopped fresh coriander
1 chopped red capsicum
1 tbspn fish sauce

Cook onion and garlic in a little lime juice on HIGH 1 minute.
Add remaining ingredients, except fish sauce, and microwave on HIGH
10 minutes.
Stir and microwave a further 10 minutes.
Add fish sauce and extra lime juice to taste, and stir through. Serves 6.

♥ approx. ·5g fat per serve

Fennel, Lemon & Thyme Risotto (Microwave)

non-stick spray
1 fennel, trimmed and sliced
1 tspn minced garlic
2 tbspns white wine
1 1/2 cups arborio rice
1 tbspn chopped fresh thyme leaves
4 cups fat-free chicken stock
2 tspns lemon rind
1 tbspn lemon juice
Native Lemon Pepper seasoning (Masterfood's brand - if unavailable use freshly ground black pepper and sea salt to taste)

Cook uncovered and use the HIGH setting for entire cooking process.
Lightly spray a large microwave-proof dish with non-stick spray. Place fennel in dish and microwave 6 minutes.
Add garlic and wine and cook further 2 minutes.
Add rice and thyme and microwave 4 minutes.
Add stock and continue cooking 9 minutes. Stir and cook further 9 minutes. Stir, then cook 4 minutes, or until nearly all the liquid is absorbed.
Add lemon rind, lemon juice and pepper to taste. Serves 4.

♥ approx. ·5g fat per serve

Tofu Vegetable Loaf

1 onion, very finely chopped
1 x 375g packet firm tofu, mashed
1 carrot, grated
1/2 cup chopped mushrooms
1/2 tspn black pepper
1/2 cup fresh breadcrumbs
1/2 tspn Worcestershire sauce
3 egg whites or substitute
1/3 cup tomato paste
1/4 tspn mustard
Tabasco sauce to taste
dash of Liquid Smoke* (optional)

Preheat oven to 180°C. Line a non-stick loaf tin with baking paper. Combine all ingredients and pour into the prepared loaf tin. Bake 45 minutes. Serves 4.

♥ approx. 1·5g fat per serve

Pumpkin, Spinach & Cottage Cheese Tart

1 large pitta bread (fat-free)
1 cup low-fat cottage cheese
400g Japanese pumpkin
100g spinach leaves, chopped
2 tbspns sweet chilli sauce
2 tspns currants
1/4 tspn dried rosemary leaves
1/4 tspn ground cinnamon
course sea salt
sesame seeds (optional)

Preheat oven to 180°C.
Place pitta bread in a pie plate. Spread cottage cheese on base of pitta.
Set aside.
Cut pumpkin into 2.5 cm cubes. Steam (or microwave for
approximately 6 minutes) until just tender.
Place on a lined oven tray and bake for 25 minutes, or until it starts to
brown on the edges.
Meanwhile, steam or microwave the spinach until it is just wilted. Place
in a bowl with the pumpkin, and add chilli sauce, currants, rosemary,
cinnamon and salt. Toss carefully so as not to break up pumpkin.
Place pumpkin mixture evenly over cheese. Sprinkle with extra sea salt
and sesame seeds. Bake 20 minutes. Serves 4.

♥ approx. 2·5g fat per serve

Pineapple Vegetable Curry

1 onion, chopped
1 stick celery, chopped
1 tspn minced garlic
2 tbspns curry paste* (oil-free)
1 cup skim milk
1 tspn coconut essence
2 tspns cornflour
pinch sugar
1 x 440g can crushed pineapple with juice
2 cups cooked mixed vegetables
fish sauce to taste
lime juice to taste

Cook onion, celery and garlic, curry paste in 1/4 cup water until onion is soft.
Combine milk, coconut essence, cornflour and sugar and add to pan.
Bring to boil, add pineapple and vegetables. Simmer covered 5 minutes, stirring occasionally.
Add fish sauce and lime juice to taste.
Serve with rice. Serves 3-4.

♥ under ·5g fat per serve

Microwave Ratatouille

2 small tomatoes, chopped
1 medium zucchini, sliced thinly
1 small eggplant, peeled and diced
1 small onion, sliced
1/2 cup green capsicum, thinly sliced
1/2 tspn minced garlic
1/2 tspn dried basil
1/4 tspn dried marjoram
1 tbspn tomato paste
salt and freshly ground black pepper
1/2 tspn parmesan cheese

Combine all ingredients in a microwave-proof casserole dish. Cover and cook on HIGH 6-8 minutes, stirring twice. Serve with crusty bread. Serves 4.

♥ neg. fat per serve

Thai Potato Cakes with Yoghurt Mint Sauce

2 cups cooked plain mashed potato
1/2 cup canned white beans, rinsed, drained and mashed
1/2 carrot grated
1 tbspn Thai curry paste* fat-free
2 egg whites or substitute
1/2 cup chopped coriander leaves
salt and freshly ground black pepper

Yoghurt Mint Sauce (page 132) to serve
mango chutney to serve

Combine all ingredients in a bowl. Place spoonfuls onto a hot non-stick fry pan and flatten with a fork. Cook until brown on each side. Serve with mango chutney and yoghurt mint sauce. Serves 2-4.

♥ under ·5g fat per serve

Moroccan Vegetables With Couscous

1/2 cup verjuice* or sweet white wine
2 large onions, cut into wedges
1 tbspn cumin powder
1 tbspn granulated garlic
2 tspns paprika
1 tspn ground cinnamon
2 zucchinis, sliced
1 x 400g can white beans, rinsed and drained
5 mushrooms, sliced
2 tbspns chopped raisins
1 cup fat-free chicken stock
4 cups diced fresh tomatoes (or use canned)
4 tbspns tomato paste
2 tspns sugar or Splenda
sea salt and pepper to taste
1 1/2 cups couscous cooked as per directions, to serve

Heat 1/4 cup verjuice in a large stockpot and cook onion, cumin, garlic and paprika 3-4 minutes.
Reduce heat and add cinnamon and more verjuice.
Add zucchini, beans, mushrooms and raisins, and stir.
Add stock, tomatoes, tomato paste and sugar or Splenda and stir through.
Bring to the boil then reduce heat, cover and simmer 15 minutes, stirring occasionally.
Uncover and cook on low heat 10 minutes more. Serve over couscous.
Serves 4-6.

♥ approx. 1·5g fat per serve

Spiced Chickpea Cakes

1 x 420g can chickpeas, rinsed and drained
1 onion, very finely chopped
1 carrot, grated
1 stick celery, very finely chopped
1/2 tspn minced garlic
1/4 tspn chilli powder
1 tspn ground cumin
1/2 cup low-fat cottage cheese
1 cup fresh breadcrumbs
1/2 tspn sumac*

Process chickpeas in a food processor then add spices and cottage cheese and process until the mixture is smooth.
Place remaining ingredients in a mixing bowl and combine with chickpea mixture.
Form into desired number of round patties and cook on a non-stick pan until browned on both sides. Serves 4.

♥ approx. 2·5g fat per serve

Ultra Quick Curry

1 small brown onion, chopped
1 small red capsicum, chopped
1 medium carrot, chopped
1 small zucchini, sliced
3 cups cooked cubed potato
1 cup pineapple pieces, drained with juice reserved
1 x 375ml can evaporated low-fat milk
1 tspn coconut essence
1 1/2 tspns cornflour
3/4 cup bean shoots
1/3 cup chopped fresh coriander leaves
2 tspns lime juice
2 tspns fish sauce
2 tbspns curry paste* (oil-free)

Place onion, capsicum, carrot, zucchini, potato and 1 cup pineapple pieces in a wok in 1/4 cup reserved pineapple juice. Stir over medium heat for 3 minutes.
Add remaining pineapple juice and cook vegetables until tender.
Combine milk, coconut essence and cornflour thoroughly and add to pan and stir until sauce thickens.
Add remaining ingredients. Serve immediately on rice or couscous.
Serves 4-6.

♥ approx. 1·5g fat per serve

Sweetcorn Pancakes with Lemongrass & Chilli

1 1/2 cups self-raising flour
3 spring onions, chopped
1/2 tspn salt
1 tspn minced garlic
1/4 tspn dried lemongrass powder
1/8 tspn chilli powder
4 egg whites or substitute
2 tbspns sweet chilli sauce
1 cup plain non-fat yoghurt
1/2 cup skim milk
1 x 425g can corn kernels, drained
squeeze lemon juice

Combine all ingredients and cook spoonfuls on a non-stick pan. When top starts to bubble, turn over carefully and cook until golden brown. Makes 8-10.

♥ under 1g fat per pancake

Savoury Vegetable Loaf

1 cup peas (fresh or frozen)
3/4 cup finely chopped onion
3 tspns water
1/4 tspn ground cloves
1 tspn freshly minced ginger
1/8 tspn five-spice powder
1 tspn dried parsley
1 tspn dried sage
1 tspn dried thyme
1 tspn dried rosemary leaves
1/4 tspn pepper
pinch salt
1 lightly packed cup grated carrot
1 1/2 cups rolled oats
1/2 cup plain non-fat yoghurt
5 egg whites or substitute
1/2 cup corn relish

Preheat oven to 180°C. Line a loaf tin with baking paper.
Combine peas, onion and water in a small saucepan and cook gently until onion is soft (or microwave for 3 minutes on HIGH).
Place onion in a mixing bowl and add remaining ingredients. Mix well.
Spoon into lined loaf tin and bake for approximately 1 hour and 25 minutes. Serves 6.

♥ approx. 3·5g fat per serve

Asparagus, Tomato & Herb Couscous

1 1/3 cups couscous
1/2 red onion, peeled and finely chopped
boiling water
1 tspn minced garlic
1 bunch asparagus, trimmed and quartered
1 tspn coriander seeds, crushed
3 cups chopped tomato
2 tbspns capers, chopped
3 tbspns lemon juice
1/2 cup chopped coriander leaves
1/2 cup chopped mint leaves
1/2 cup chopped parsley
1/4 cup chopped chives
sea salt and freshly ground black pepper

Combine couscous and onion in a casserole dish. Pour enough boiling hot water over the top to cover the couscous. Stir then cover dish and set aside for 10 minutes.
Place garlic in a large saucepan with 1 tbspn water and cook 1 minute. Add asparagus and coriander seeds and cook 1 minute.
Add couscous and stir through gently.
Add tomatoes, capers, lemon juice, and chopped herbs and cook until couscous is heated through.
Serve with salt and pepper to taste. Serves 4.

♥ approx. 1g fat per serve

Spiced Couscous with Chickpeas & Asparagus Sauce

spiced couscous:
1 cup couscous
1 tspn chicken stock powder
1/2 brown onion, chopped
1 tbspn chopped fresh thyme leaves
white wine
2 tspns cumin seeds
2 tbspns chopped fresh coriander leaves
sea salt and freshly ground black pepper

sauce:
1 bunch asparagus, cut into quarters
1 x 400g can chickpeas, rinsed and drained
1 tspn minced garlic
1 tspn chilli powder
1 tbspn sweet chilli sauce
3 tbspns low fat ricotta cheese
1/2 cup vegetable stock

Place couscous and stock powder in a bowl and pour 1 1/2 cups boiling water over. Stir, cover and stand 10 minutes.
Cook onion and thyme in a little wine until soft and then add cumin seeds, coriander leaves, salt and pepper. Add extra wine as necessary. Stir through the couscous.
Cook asparagus and chickpeas together in a pan for 1 minute and then add garlic, chilli powder, chilli sauce, ricotta and stock to the pan. Cook until sauce forms and mixture is heated through. Serve over the couscous with extra chilli sauce to taste.

♥ approx. 2·5g fat per serve

Lentil Dhal (Microwave)

250g red lentils, washed and picked over
1 tbspn curry powder
1 tspn salt
1/2 tspn turmeric
4 cups hot water
1 carrot, diced
1 large onion, chopped
4 tomatoes, chopped
1/4 cup tomato paste
1/4 tspn chilli flakes (optional)
1 tspn garam masala
2 tbspns lemon juice

Place lentils, curry powder, salt, turmeric and 2 cups water in a large microwave safe casserole dish. Cook 10 minutes HIGH.
Stir and add another 1 cup water. Cook further 5 minutes.
Stir; add diced carrot and final cup hot water. Cook 5 minutes HIGH.
Place the onion, tomatoes, tomato paste, chilli flakes and a little water in a non-stick pan over a hotplate. Cover and cook until onion soft and transparent, adding a little extra water if necessary.
Add lentils and stir to heat through. Add lemon juice and garam masala. Stir into mixture and serve with pita bread and basmati rice.
Serves 4.

♥ approx. 1·5g fat per serve

Potato, Chickpea & Green Bean Curry (Microwave)

1/2 tspn minced garlic
2 coriander roots, washed
1/2 tspn whole black peppercorns
1 tbspn water
1 tbspn curry powder
1 x 375 tin evaporated low-fat milk
2 tspns cornflour
1 tspn coconut essence
2 cooked potatoes
1 x 400g can chickpeas, rinsed and drained
1 cup frozen green beans, thawed and drained
2 large tomatoes, chopped
1 tbspn basil leaves
1 tbspn coriander leaves
2-3 tbspns soy sauce
1/2 tspn salt
1 tspn sugar or Splenda

Place garlic, coriander roots and peppercorns in a mortar and pestle. Grind until crushed and paste-like.
Place the mixture in a microwave-proof dish with 1 tspn water and microwave covered HIGH for 30 seconds.
Add curry powder and cook further 30 seconds.
In a jug, thoroughly combine evaporated milk with cornflour and essence and then add to dish. Stir through and microwave uncovered for 1 minute.
Cut the cooked potatoes into 2 cm cubes and add to dish with chickpeas and beans. Stirring every minute, microwave uncovered for 4 minutes.
Add tomato, basil, coriander, soy sauce, salt and sugar. Cover and microwave 2 minutes. Stir and then cook further 2 minutes.
Check for seasoning and serve over rice. Serves 4.

♥ approx. 2·5g fat per serve

Mustard Potato Patties

4 medium potatoes, cooked and mashed
1/3 cup corn kernels
2 tbspns seeded mustard
1/3 cup chopped fresh parsley
2 tbspns hot English mustard
2 tbspns skim milk

Combine all ingredients. Shape mixture into patties.
Cook on a non-stick grill plate or pan, until brown on each side.
Serves 4.

♥ approx. ·5g fat per serve

Autumn Vegetable Medley

1 onion, finely diced
1 tspn minced garlic
1/4 tspn ground coriander
1/4 tspn cumin powder
1/4 tspn paprika
1/4 tspn cayenne pepper
1 small eggplant, diced
1 red capsicum, diced
1 cup corn kernels
1 zucchini, diced
2 large ripe tomatoes
salt and freshly ground black pepper to taste
3 tbspns yoghurt cheese (page 138)
3 tbspns chopped fresh coriander leaves

Cook onion on low-medium heat in 1 tbspn water in a non-stick wok until soft. Add garlic and spices. Stir.
Add eggplant and capsicum. Cook gently, stirring often.
Add corn kernels, zucchini and tomatoes. Continue cooking. Season with salt and pepper, add yoghurt cheese and stir through until combined and heated through.
Add coriander and serve over couscous or rice. Serves 4.

♥ approx. ·5g fat per serve

Chickpea & Vegetable Mix

2 medium potatoes, peeled and diced
1 x 425g can chickpeas, rinsed and drained
1 tspn minced garlic
2 tspns dried thyme leaves
1/2 tspn dried chilli flakes
1 tbspn capers
2 medium carrots, sliced
500g fresh chopped tomatoes or 1 x 400g canned
3 cups fat-free chicken stock
1 small zucchini, sliced
5-6 mushrooms, quartered
1/3 cup chopped parsley

Steam, boil or microwave potatoes until tender.
Add cooked potatoes to a large saucepan with chickpeas, garlic, thyme, chilli flakes, capers, carrots, tomatoes and stock. Bring to the boil. Simmer uncovered 10 minutes.
Add zucchini and mushrooms and cook further 10 minutes. Stir through the parsley. Serve on couscous. Serves 4.

♥ approx. 1·5g fat per serve (without couscous)

Notes

Notes

Living Lite

salads &
side vegetables

Photo right: *Sweet Carrots (page 99), Savoury Wheat Salad (page 90), Balsamic Asparagus (page 94), Pizza Potatoes (page 98)*

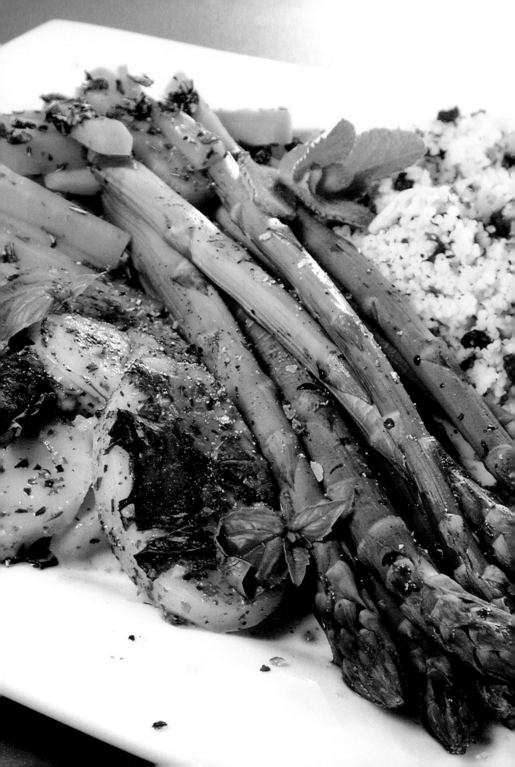

Chicken & Vegetable Salad
with Spicy Lime Dressing

5 sun-dried tomatoes, (not in oil)
2 x 125g chicken breast fillets, skinned and all visible fat removed
1 1/2 cups snow peas, halved
300g macaroni, cooked and well drained
1 large carrot, sliced thinly
1 small red capsicum, chopped
3 cups sliced mushrooms
4 spring onions, chopped

Spicy Lime Dressing:
1/3 cup lime juice
1/3 cup fat-free mayonnaise (page 132) or 99% fat-free mayonnaise
(eg Kraft or Freedom Foods)
1/4 cup sweet chilli sauce
1/3 cup chopped fresh coriander

Combine dressing ingredients and set aside.
Soak sun-dried tomatoes in boiling water for 10 minutes, drain and
slice.
Slice chicken into 1·5 cm slices. Steam or microwave chicken until
cooked, drain and pat dry.
Plunge snow peas in boiling water for a minute, and then plunge into
iced water. Drain and pat dry.
Combine chicken with sun-dried tomatoes, snow peas, macaroni,
carrot, capsicum, mushrooms and spring onions.
Pour the dressing over and mix gently to combine.

♥ approx. 7·5g fat in entire salad

Thai-Style Vegetable Salad

1/2 small red onion chopped
1 small carrot, thinly sliced
1 clove garlic, crushed
2 tspns dried coriander
1/8 tspn freshly ground black pepper
2 tbspns finely chopped lemongrass
1/4 cup finely chopped mint leaves
1/4 tspn sugar
1 tbspn lime juice (or to taste)
1 tbspn soy sauce (or to taste)
1 tbspn fish sauce (or to taste)
2 tbspns chilli paste
1 tspn dried chilli
3 cups sliced mushrooms
1/4 cup baby corn
1 1/2 cups chopped lettuce
1 tbspn finely chopped unsalted peanuts (optional)
handful mixed salad sprouts
1 Lebanese cucumber, thinly sliced

garnish:
extra mint leaves
bean shoots
cucumber slices
fresh coriander leaves
torn lettuce leaves

Spray a non-stick pan or wok with non-stick spray.
Add onion and carrot and stir-fry 1 minute.
Add garlic, dried coriander, pepper, lemon grass, mint, sugar, lime juice, soy sauce, fish sauce, chilli paste and dried chilli. Cook 2 minutes.
Add mushrooms, corn, lettuce, peanuts, salad sprouts and cucumber. Cook further 2 minutes. Add extra soy sauce if necessary.
Add extra seasonings to taste. Serve with garnish ingredients.

♥ approx. 8g fat in entire salad with peanuts

Pasta Salad

250g macaroni
1/2 red capsicum, finely chopped
2 spring onions, finely sliced
5 sun-dried tomatoes, not in oil
5-6 mushrooms, sliced
2 tbspns finely chopped fresh parsley

dressing:
1 cup plain non-fat yoghurt
2 tspns tomato paste
1 tbspn lemon juice
1 tbspn orange juice
2 tspns curry powder

Cook the macaroni, drain and rinse with cold water. Leave to cool.
Meanwhile, soak the sun-dried tomatoes in hot water for 10 minutes.
Drain and dry. Slice finely.
Combine all the dressing ingredients thoroughly.
Combine the macaroni and sliced tomatoes with remaining salad
ingredients in a salad bowl and toss the dressing through to coat.

♥ approx. 4g fat in entire salad

Potato Salad

3 medium potatoes, peeled and diced
2 tbspns chopped fresh parsley
1 tbspn chopped red capsicum
1/4 cup corn kernels
3 spring onions, finely sliced
freshly ground black pepper to taste

dressing:
2 tbspns oil-free Italian dressing
1/2 cup plain non-fat yoghurt

Cook potatoes until soft but still holding shape. Drain and allow to cool.
When cool, combine with the parsley, capsicum, corn kernels and
spring onions. Season to taste with pepper.
Combine the dressing with the yoghurt and add to potato. Mix carefully
through. Chill before serving.

♥ approx.1·5g fat in entire salad

Crab & Mango Salad

1 tspn sweet chilli sauce
1 tbspn fresh lime juice
salt and freshly ground black pepper
1 x 170g can crabmeat, drained
2 tbspns chopped fresh mint
2 tbspns chopped fresh coriander
1 mango, cubed

Whisk together the chilli sauce, lime juice, salt and pepper to taste.
Combine gently with remaining ingredients.
Serve on a flat plate lined with lettuce leaves.

♥ approx. 1·5g fat in entire salad

Savoury Wheat Salad

1/2 cup burghal wheat
1 1/2 cups hot water
2-3 spring onions, finely sliced
2 tbspns currants
2 tbspns chopped fresh mint
2 tbspns chopped fresh coriander
3 tbspns oil-free French dressing
freshly ground pepper

In a small saucepan, bring the burghal wheat and water to a boil. Reduce heat and simmer, covered for 10-12 minutes, until all the moisture is absorbed.
Combine with remaining ingredients in a salad bowl and chill at least 30 minutes before serving.

♥ approx. 2g fat in entire salad

Green Bean & Apple Salad

2 cups fresh green beans, topped and tailed
2 tbspns chopped dried apple
2 pinches dried dill weed
dash of extra dill to decorate

dressing:
2 tbspns Dijon mustard
1 tbspn Balsamic vinegar
1 tbspn yoghurt cheese (page 138)
1 tspn apple juice

Blanch or steam beans and then plunge them immediately into very
cold water so they retain colour. Drain and dry thoroughly.
Whisk together the mustard, vinegar, yoghurt cheese and apple juice.
Combine beans and dried apple and stir through the dill weed.
Add the dressing and stir to cover apple and beans thoroughly.
Sprinkle a little extra dried dill over top.

♥ neg. fat in entire salad

Rice Salad

2 cups cold cooked rice
handful currants
1 tbspn chopped fresh mint
3 tbspns corn kernels
1 spring onion, chopped
2 tbspns chopped capsicum

dressing:
1/4 cup white wine vinegar
1 tbspn French mustard
dash Tabasco sauce
1 tbspn honey
salt and pepper to taste

Combine dressing ingredients in a jar and shake to incorporate
thoroughly.
Combine all salad ingredients and toss dressing through.

♥ approx. 3g fat in entire salad

Marinated Mushrooms And Artichokes

450g mushrooms, sliced in halves
1 x 400g can artichokes hearts, drained and cut in halves

marinade:
90 mls water
3 tbspns oil-free French dressing
1/4 tspn minced garlic
1/8 tspn dried thyme
2 tbspns cider vinegar
1 tspn sea salt
5 peppercorns
2 tspns chopped fresh basil
1 bay leaf
1 tbspn lemon juice

Place the mushrooms and artichokes in a dish.
Combine the marinade ingredients in a small saucepan and heat – do not
bring to the boil.
Pour over mushrooms and artichokes and refrigerate overnight.
Remove peppercorns and bay leaf before serving.

♥ neg. fat in entire dish

Balsamic Asparagus

2 bunches fresh asparagus, trimmed, left whole
balsamic vinegar
sea salt
freshly ground black pepper

Preheat oven to 250°C.
Place a roasting pan in oven for 5 minutes to heat through.
Place the asparagus in the hot pan. Return to oven and roast 5 minutes
or until just tender.
Remove pan from oven and sprinkle a little balsamic vinegar, sea salt
and freshly ground black pepper over the asparagus.

♥ neg. fat in entire dish

Eggplant With Herbs (Microwave)

2 small eggplants
1/4 tspn minced garlic
2 tspns thyme leaves
2 tspns lemon juice
1/2 tspn ground coriander
freshly ground black pepper
pinch sea salt
1/4 cup chopped red capsicum

Wash eggplants and prick all over with a fork. Microwave 5 minutes on
HIGH, turning halfway during the cooking. Wrap in paper towel and set
aside.
Place remaining ingredients in a microwave proof dish and cook 1
minute HIGH.
Slice eggplants into medallions and add to other ingredients. Delicious
served over mashed potato.

♥ neg. fat in entire dish

Lime & Dill Potato Puree

2 medium Desiree potatoes, peeled and chopped
pinch sea salt
grated rind 1 lime
lime juice of 1 lime
1/4 tspn cumin powder
1/4 tspn dried dill
skim milk

Cook, drain and mash potatoes.
Add salt, lime juice, lime rind, cumin powder and dill and mix through.
Add enough skim milk to make a creamy consistency.
This is delicious served under grilled salmon or tuna steaks.

♥ neg. fat in entire dish

Dill Cabbage

1 medium onion, chopped
1 tbspn white wine
3 tbspns lemon juice
1 tspn dried dill
2 tbspns chopped dried apple
1/8 tspn white pepper
2 cups shredded cabbage
1 tbspn Dijon mustard
2 extra tbspns lemon juice

Place onion, wine, lemon juice, dill and dried apple in a medium saucepan and cook (or microwave 3-4 minutes) until onion is transparent.
Add pepper, cabbage, mustard and extra lemon juice.
Cook (or microwave 4 minutes) until cabbage is soft.

♥ neg. fat in entire dish

Pizza Potatoes (Microwave)

2 small whole potatoes, cooked
1/2 cup evaporated low-fat milk
1 tspn cornflour
2 tspns Pizza Topper seasoning (Masterfood's brand)
6 leaves basil, torn

Slice the potatoes into desirable sized slices.
Combine the milk and cornflour thoroughly.
Add Pizza Topper seasoning and basil and stir through until blended.
Pour over potatoes and gently mix through taking care not to break up the potato.
Microwave 1-2 minutes, stirring halfway through cooking time. Serves 2.

♥ approx. 1g fat per serve

Sweet Carrots

4 carrots, peeled and sliced
2 tspns honey
1/2 tspn dried rosemary
1 tbspn freshly chopped mint

Steam or microwave carrots and drain.
Drizzle honey over top of carrots and stir through rosemary and mint.
Reheat if necessary. Serves 4 as a side vegetable.

♥ neg. fat in entire dish

Fennel in Herbs & White Wine

1 fennel bulb, trimmed and sliced
good squeeze lemon juice
1/4 tspn grated lemon rind
pinch sea salt and freshly ground black pepper
1 tspn chopped fresh thyme leaves
1 tbspn chopped fresh rosemary leaves
1 tspn chopped fresh sage leaves
1 tbspn chopped fresh parsley
1/4 cup fat-free chicken stock
2 tspns chopped capers
1/4 cup white wine

Combine all ingredients in a saucepan and cook over medium heat until comes it to the boil (or microwave 12-15 minutes).
Lower heat and simmer until soft, approximately 30 minutes (or microwave further 10 minutes). Serves 4 as a side vegetable.

♥ neg. fat in entire dish

Pumpkin Risotto Cakes

350g Japanese pumpkin, peeled and chopped
1 tspn Parmesan cheese
4 1/2 cups fat-free chicken stock
1 cup dry white wine
1 onion, chopped
2 cups arborio rice
freshly ground black pepper

Preheat oven to 180°C.
Place pumpkin on an oven tray lined with baking paper. Bake 25 minutes. Mash cooked pumpkin with the parmesan cheese.
In a saucepan, combine 4 cups of the chicken stock and 3/4 cup of the wine and heat over medium heat.
In a separate pot, heat remaining 1/2 cup stock. Add the onion and cook until soft and almost all liquid absorbed.
Add rice to the onion, stir very quickly to toast the rice, then add remaining 1/4 cup wine and stir 1-2 minutes.
Add hot stock to rice, 1 cup at a time, stirring continuously until all liquid absorbed.
Remove from heat. Add mashed pumpkin. Let stand 10 minutes. Shape into patties and dry fry. Serves 6.

♥ approx. ·5g fat per serve

Lite & Easy Vegetable Combinations

These very simple combinations of ingredients can be cooked as side vegetables. Serve them with fish, chicken or other vegetarian dishes. Cook them however you wish – microwave, steam or stir-fry and vary amounts to suit your own taste. Vegetables contain virtually no fat.

♥ Sliced leeks cooked in balsamic vinegar, with sumac* and torn fresh basil leaves.

♥ Sliced spring onions, cracked pepper, chopped raisins, sliced mushrooms and soy sauce.

♥ Mashed cooked potato with chopped fresh sage leaves, ground coriander, parsley, salt and pepper, ricotta cheese and skim milk.

♥ Mashed cooked potato with chopped spring onions, nutmeg, salt and freshly ground black pepper, lemon juice and skim milk.

♥ Sliced mushrooms, soy sauce, freshly ground black pepper, basil, spring onions, verjuice* (cook in a foil pan on the barbecue).

♥ Dry-fry 1/2 tspn coriander seeds in a non-stick pan and then cook with thinly sliced zucchini, chopped capers, plain non-fat yoghurt, and a pinch ground coriander.

♥ Grated zucchini with mint, parsley, lemon slices and white wine vinegar.

♥ Eggplant (first, prick with a fork, and cook whole in oven or microwave until soft), sliced and cooked with capers, oregano, mint and lemon juice.

♥ Sliced carrots cooked in chicken stock, chopped raisins, parsley and ground coriander.

♥ Fresh asparagus cooked with sliced mushrooms, soy sauce, chilli flakes and a good sprinkle of dried tarragon.

♥ Sliced zucchini, capsicum, spring onions, cooked in lemon juice, lemon rind, freshly ground black pepper and pre-soaked sun-dried tomatoes (not in oil).

Living Lite

biscuits, cakes & muffins

Photo right: *Rum & Raisin Chocolate Supreme*
(recipe page 116)

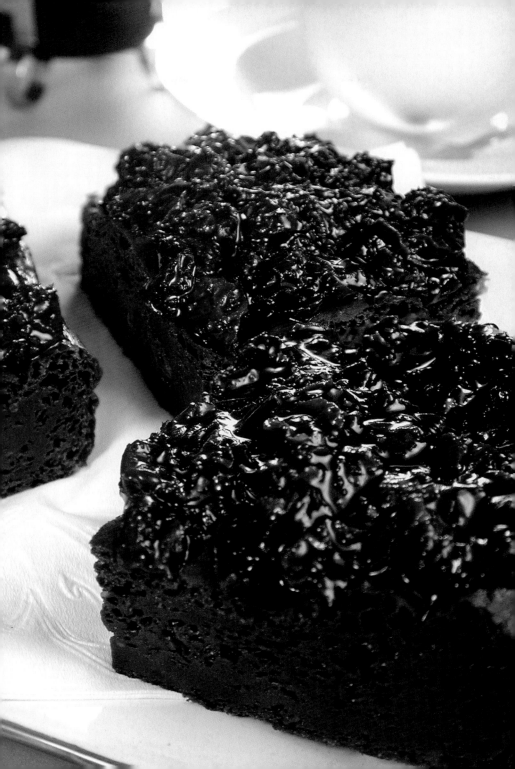

Anzac Biscuits

My son loves his Nanna's homemade Anzac biscuits so I set out to cut the fat and sugar from the traditional recipe. I devised this recipe and my son couldn't tell the difference. They still contain some fat and sugar, but I managed to reduce the fat content from around 4g to around 1.5g per biscuit, and the calorie value from 129 down to around 46!

1/2 cup plain flour
1/2 cup wholemeal plain flour
1 cup rolled oats
2 tbspns desiccated coconut
1/2 cup white sugar
1/2 cup Splenda
65g polyunsaturated margarine
65g fat replacer*
2 tbspns pancake syrup (Karo brand)
1/2 tspn baking soda
1 tbspn boiling water

Preheat oven to 150°C. Line 2 biscuit trays with baking paper.
Sift flours into a bowl. Add oats, coconut, sugar and Splenda.
Combine margarine, fat replacer and pancake syrup and stir over low heat until melted (or microwave 20 seconds). Remove from heat.
Combine baking soda with boiling water and add to the butter mixture.
Stir this mixture into the dry ingredients.
Spoon mixture onto lined biscuit trays to make 48 biscuits. Cook 10-15 minutes. Loosen biscuits while warm, and then leave to cool on trays.

♥ approx. 1·5g fat per biscuit

Cornflake Cookies

1 cup white self-raising flour
1/4 cup sugar or Splenda
1/4 tspn salt
1/2 tspn bicarb of soda
1 tspn mixed spice
1/4 tspn nutmeg
1 cup cornflakes lightly crushed
1/2 cup currants
2 egg whites or substitute*
1/3 cup rice syrup*
1 tspn vanilla essence
baking glaze (page 135)

Preheat oven to 175°C. Line a non-stick oven tray with baking paper.
Sift first six ingredients. Add cornflakes and currants.
Combine egg whites, rice syrup and essence. Add to dry ingredients.
Working quickly with damp hands (the mixture will be very sticky) form
the mixture into 15 biscuits. Bake 10 minutes.
Remove from oven and brush lightly with baking glaze. Bake further 10
minutes.
Remove from trays immediately and cool on cake rack.

♥ neg. fat per cookie

Chocolate Brownies

1/3 cup cocoa powder
2/3 cup self-raising flour
1/2 tspn bicarb of soda
1/8 tspn salt
1/3 cup sugar
1/3 cup Splenda
1/3 cup orange juice
1/3 cup skim milk
1/3 cup prune puree*
1 1/2 tspns vanilla essence
2 egg whites or substitute*

Preheat oven to 160°C. Line a non-stick 20cm square cake pan with baking paper.
Sift cocoa powder, flour, bicarb and salt into a mixing bowl. Add sugar and Splenda and mix through.
Separately combine orange juice, milk, prune puree, vanilla essence and egg whites in a bowl or jug and mix thoroughly.
Add wet ingredients to dry ingredients and mix well.
Pour into cake pan. Bake 30-35 minutes. Test centre with a skewer.
Leave to cool in cake pan 10 minutes before inverting onto a chopping board.
Let cool completely before cutting into 16 squares. Dust with icing sugar and cocoa powder if desired.

♥ under 1g fat per brownie

Lemon & Poppy Seed Muffins

1 3/4 cups self-raising flour
1 tspn baking powder
1/3 cup sugar or Splenda
1 tbspn poppy seeds
1 tbspn grated lemon rind
1/4 cup commercial apple sauce or Apple Puree (page 131)
1 cup skim milk
2 egg whites or substitute*
1 tbspn lemon juice

Preheat oven to 190°C.
Sift flour and baking powder together into a bowl. Add sugar or Splenda and poppy seeds.
Combine remaining ingredients and add to bowl. Mix with a wooden spoon until just combined – do not over mix.
Spoon mixture into a 12-cup muffin tin. Bake 12-15 minutes. Makes 12.

♥ under 1g fat per muffin

Banana Maple Date Muffins

This recipe makes 12 normal size muffins or 6 jumbo muffins (extend cooking time by 5 minutes for 6).

1 cup wholemeal self-raising flour
1 cup white self-raising flour
3 tbspns sugar or Splenda
1 cup chopped dates
3 ripe bananas, mashed
1/2 cup evaporated low-fat milk
1/4 cup maple syrup
2 egg whites or substitute*

Preheat oven to 175°C.
Combine flours, sugar or Splenda and dates in a mixing bowl.
Combine banana, milk, maple syrup and egg whites in a separate bowl.
Add the wet ingredients to the dry ingredients and mix to combine but do not over-mix.
Spoon into a non-stick muffin tray.
Bake for 15-18 minutes. Let muffins stand 5 minutes before removing from tin to cool on a wire cake rack.

♥ 6 muffins - approx. 1·5g fat per muffin
♥ 12 muffins - approx. ·6g fat per muffin

Rock Cakes

1 cup plain wholemeal flour
1 cup plain white flour
2 tspns baking powder
2/3 cup sugar or Splenda
1/2 cup sultanas
1/3 cup mixed peel
2 tspns grated lemon rind
1/4 cup commercial apple sauce or Apple Puree (page 131)
140mls skim milk (approx)
1 tbspn diet vanilla yoghurt

Preheat oven to 200°C. Line a non-stick oven tray with baking paper.
Sift flours and baking powder into a mixing bowl.
Add sugar or Splenda, sultanas, peel and lemon rind.
Combine apple puree, milk and yoghurt together and add to flour.
Mix to form a tacky dough. Drop 12 roughly shaped cakes onto tray.
Bake in preheated oven for 20 minutes. Cool on a cake rack.

♥ approx. ·5g fat each

Fruity Spiral Buns

pastry:
2/3 cup self-raising flour
2 tbspns sugar or Splenda
1/8 tspn cinnamon
1/2 cup plain non-fat yoghurt

filling:
2 tbspns marmalade or apricot jam (no added sugar)
1/4 cup sultanas
5 dried Turkish apricots, sliced
pinch mixed spice
extra jam or marmalade to glaze

Preheat oven to 175°C.
Combine flour, sugar and cinnamon in a mixing bowl. Add yoghurt and mix to form a soft dough. Turn out onto floured pastry board and very gently form a ball. Roll out into a rectangle (roughly 30cm X 12cm). With a knife, gently spread marmalade or jam over full surface of dough. Arrange sultanas and apricots evenly over top. Sprinkle with mixed spice.
Roll pastry up into a long log shape. With a floured sharp knife, slice into 6 equal pieces. Arrange onto a lined non-stick tray fruit filling sides up. Bake 15 minutes.
Remove from oven and brush with jam or marmalade. Bake further 8 minutes. Place on cake rack to cool.

♥ approx. ·5g fat each

Christmas Fruit Slice

1 cup rolled oats
1/4 cup sultanas
1/4 cup currants
1 cup chopped dried apricots
12 glace cherries chopped
1/2 tspn cinnamon
1/8 tspn ground cloves
1/8 tspn nutmeg
1/4 tspn mixed spice
1 cup sweetened condensed skim milk
4 egg whites or substitute*
1/3 cup fat free fruit mince*
1 tspn vanilla essence

Preheat oven to 150°C.
Combine all ingredients. Pour into a lined square cake tin. Bake for 1 to
1 1/4 hours.
Cool in tin and when cool, cut into 16 slices.

♥ approx. 1g fat per slice

Maple And Pear Cake

1 x 425g tin pear halves with juice
3/4 cup rolled oats
1/4 cup processed bran
3/4 cup sultanas
1/3 cup maple syrup
3 tbspns sugar or Splenda
1 1/2 cups wholemeal self-raising flour
1 tspn baking powder
1/2 cup diet vanilla yoghurt

topping (optional):
1 cup icing sugar, sifted
1 tbspn diet vanilla yoghurt
2 tspns maple syrup
water as required

Dice pear halves. Combine with juice, oats, bran, sultanas, maple syrup and sugar or Splenda and let stand for 2 hours.
Preheat oven to 175°C.
Add flour, baking powder and yoghurt to the pear mixture. Mix thoroughly but do not beat.
Spoon mixture into a non-stick round or square cake pan (18 cm).
Bake 40-45 minutes. Cool in pan 10 minutes, then transfer to a wire cake rack to cool completely.
When cold, ice with topping if desired.
To make topping, mix icing sugar, yoghurt and maple syrup thoroughly. Add a little water to mixture as required until mixture is desired consistency.

♥ approx. 13g fat in entire cake (including topping)

Carrot Cake

2 cups wholemeal self-raising flour
1 tspn baking powder
1 tspn cinnamon
1 tspn mixed spice
1/8 tspn nutmeg
1/8 tspn salt
2 cups grated carrot
1 cup sultanas
1/2 cup sugar or Splenda
1/2 cup plain non-fat yoghurt
4 egg whites or substitute*
2 tspn vanilla essence
1/2 cup apple juice concentrate*
1/4 cup apple juice

frosting:
rind of one lemon
3/4 cup low-fat ricotta cheese
1/4 tspn lemon essence
1 tbspn apple juice concentrate*

Preheat oven to 180°C.
Sift flour, baking powder, spices and salt into a mixing bowl.
Separately combine carrot, sultanas, sugar, yoghurt, egg whites, essence,
apple juice concentrate and apple juice.
Add wet ingredients to flour mixture.
Mix well and spoon into a large non-stick pan. Bake 30 minutes. Invert
onto a cake rack to cool completely.
Combine frosting ingredients and spread over cooled cake.

♥ approx. 13g fat in entire cake (including frosting)

Easy Banana Cake

(pictured on front cover, top right)

4 egg whites or substitute*
1/2 cup sugar or Splenda
4 ripe bananas, mashed
1/2 cup diet vanilla yoghurt
2 tbspns skim milk powder
1 cup chopped dates
1 cup wholemeal self-raising flour
1 cup white self-raising flour
1/4 tspn salt
1 tspn bicarb of soda

frosting:
rind of one lemon
3/4 cup low-fat ricotta cheese
1/4 tspn lemon essence
1 tbspn apple juice concentrate*

Preheat oven to 180°C. Line a non-stick loaf cake pan with baking paper.
Combine the egg whites, sugar or Splenda, mashed banana, yoghurt and milk powder in a large mixing bowl. Add the dates and stir through.
Sift the flours, salt and bicarb of soda into a separate bowl.
Add sifted dry ingredients to banana mixture.
Spoon into prepared loaf pan. Bake 40-45 minutes or until skewer inserted into centre of cake comes out clean.
Remove from pan to cool on a cake rack.
When cake is cool, combine frosting ingredients and spread over cake.

♥ approx. 15g fat in entire cake (including frosting)

Rum And Raisin Chocolate Supreme

1 cup self-raising flour
1/4 cup cocoa powder
1 tspn bicarb of soda
3/4 cup Splenda
1/3 cup chopped raisins
1/2 cup commercial apple sauce or Apple Puree (page 131)
2 egg whites or substitute*
1 cup plain non-fat yoghurt
1 tbspn skim milk powder
1 tbspn rum

topping:
1/2 cup chopped raisins
1/4 cup apple juice
1 tbspn rum
1 tbspn cocoa powder
1 sachet powdered sweetener

Preheat oven to 180°C. Line a 20 cm square non-stick cake pan with baking paper.
Sift flour, cocoa powder and bicarb of soda into a bowl. Add Splenda and raisins and combine thoroughly.
Combine apple puree, egg whites, yoghurt, milk powder and rum in a bowl and then add to flour mixture. Mix until well combined.
Spoon into cake pan and bake for 30-35 minutes. Allow cake to cool in the pan and then invert onto cake rack. Spread with topping.

To make topping:
Combine raisins, apple juice and rum in a small saucepan and bring to the boil. Simmer until almost all but roughly one teaspoon of the liquid is absorbed.
Remove from heat and stir through the cocoa powder and sweetener. Let cool before spreading onto cake.

♥ approx. 15g fat in entire cake

Notes

Notes

Living Lite

desserts

Photo right: *Chocolate Pudding*
(recipe page 122)

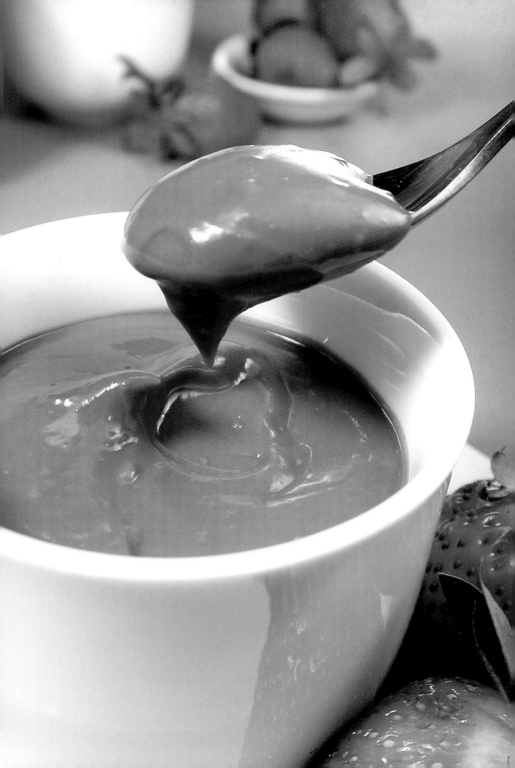

Caramel Cheesecake

base:
1 1/4 cups Nutrigrain
1/3 cup cornflake crumbs
2 tbspns sugar or Splenda
2 egg whites or substitute*

filling:
200g low-fat ricotta cheese or quark*
200g low-fat cottage cheese
3/4 cup low-fat vanilla yoghurt
1/2 cup diet caramel topping (Cottees)
3 tspns gelatine
3 tbspns boiling water

Preheat oven to 180°C. Spray a 23cm pie plate with non-stick spray. Process Nutrigrain in a food processor until it is crumbly. Add cornflakes and sugar or Splenda and process briefly. Add egg whites and process again until mixture is combined. Remove from processor and press evenly into pie plate. Bake 7 minutes.
Blend ricotta (or quark) and cottage cheese in a food processor until smooth.
Add yoghurt and caramel topping and blend again.
Sprinkle gelatine over boiling water and dissolve thoroughly. Add to mixture and process again to combine.
Pour into base and refrigerate to set for at least 4 hours. Serves 8.

♥ approx. 2g fat per serve

Lemon Cheesecake

base:
1 cup Nutrigrain
1/4 cup cornflake crumbs
1 1/2 tbspns apple juice concentrate*

filling:
1 1/4 cup low-fat cottage cheese
1 cup low-fat vanilla yoghurt
3 tbspns lemon juice
2 tspns lemon rind
1 tspn vanilla essence
5 tbspns sugar or Splenda
1 tbspn gelatine
2 tbspns boiling water

Place Nutrigrain in a food processor and process until crumbly. Add cornflakes and apple juice concentrate and process further until the mixture forms a grainy texture. Press into a 28cm round pie plate lined with plastic wrap to form a firm base and place in a freezer until the filling is ready.
Place yoghurt, cottage cheese, lemon juice, lemon rind, essence and sugar or Splenda in a food processor and process until smooth.
Dissolve gelatine in boiling water and stir. Set aside to cool a little, and then add to processor, while processor is running, until well blended. Pour into base. Refrigerate for at least 2 hours to set. Serves 8.

♥ approx. 2g fat per serve

Roasted Pears with Vanilla Spiced Yoghurt

(pictured on front cover, bottom right)

4-5 firm ripe pears, washed
2 tbspns freshly squeezed lemon juice
2 tbspns soft brown sugar

Vanilla Spiced Yoghurt:
1 x 200ml tub diet vanilla yoghurt
1 heaped 1/4 tspn ground cinnamon
1 heaped 1/4 tspn ground ginger

Preheat oven to 200°C.
Slice pears into quarters lengthways and remove core, leaving stem intact.
Place into a shallow ovenproof baking tray and sprinkle evenly with lemon juice and the sugar. Bake 30 minutes, gently turning every 10 minutes.
Serve hot, warm or cold with vanilla spiced yoghurt.
To make yoghurt, combine all ingredients thoroughly. Serves 4.

♥ approx. ·5g fat per serve

Chocolate Pudding

4 tbspns drinking chocolate powder
4 tbspns cornflour
2 cups skim milk
1 tbspn sugar or Splenda
1 tspn vanilla essence

Sift the drinking chocolate and cornflour into a medium saucepan.
Gradually stir in the milk and stir until dissolved.
Add sugar or Splenda and cook over medium heat, stirring continuously until thick and smooth.
Remove from heat, add vanilla essence and stir through.
Pour immediately into 4 dessert bowls and refrigerate.
Serve with any of the sweet sauces or toppings (pages 133-134) if desired. Serves 4.

♥ under 1g fat per serve

Apricot, Lemon & Banana Fruit Pie

(pictured on front cover, bottom right)

1 1/4 cups low-fat cottage cheese
1 x 400g can apricot halves in natural juice
1 banana, roughly chopped
1/2 cup sugar or Splenda
1/2 cup custard powder
grated lemon rind of 1 lemon
6 egg whites or substitute*
1 tspn coconut essence

Preheat oven to 180°C.
Blend all ingredients in a food processor until smooth.
Pour into a lightly sprayed 20cm pie plate. Bake 30-40 minutes. Serve warm.
Serve with Citrus Cream (page 134) if desired.Serves 8.

♥ approx. 1·5g fat per serve

Fruit Juice Flan

base:
1 1/4 cups Nutrigrain
1/3 cup cornflake crumbs
2 tbspns apple juice concentrate*

filling:
2 1/2 cups dark grape juice
2/3 cup sugar or Splenda
4 1/2 tbspns cornflour
1/4 tspn salt
1 tspn finely grated lemon rind
1/2 tspn ground cinnamon
3 tspns fresh lemon juice
strawberries to decorate

Place Nutrigrain in a food processor and process until crumbly. Add cornflakes and apple juice concentrate and process further until the mixture forms a grainy texture. Press into a 23cm round pie plate lined with plastic wrap. This will make it easier to lift whole dessert out if desired. Place in freezer until filling is ready.

Place grape juice, sugar or Splenda, cornflour, salt, lemon rind and cinnamon in a saucepan. Whisk to ensure all ingredients are thoroughly combined. Stir with a spoon over low heat until mixture becomes a very thick syrup consistency and coats the back of the spoon. Remove from heat and add lemon juice. Combine thoroughly. Let cool.

Pour into prepared base and refrigerate to set. Decorate with strawberries to serve.

Serve with Sweet Maple Cinnamon Sauce (page 133) if desired. Serves 6.

♥ approx. ·5g fat per serve

Baked Banana Maple Pie

base:
1 1/4 cups Nutrigrain
1/3 cup cornflake crumbs
2 tbspns sugar or Splenda
2 egg whites or substitute*

filling:
2 ripe bananas, roughly chopped
1/2 cup low-fat ricotta cheese
1 tspn vanilla essence
1 tbspn maple syrup
4 egg whites or substitute*
3/4 cup evaporated low-fat milk

Preheat oven to 180°C. Spray a 23cm pie plate with non-stick spray. Process Nutrigrain in a food processor until it is crumbly. Add cornflakes and Splenda and process briefly. Add the 2 egg whites and process again until mixture is combined. Remove from processor and press evenly into pie plate. Bake for 7 minutes.
To make the filling, process bananas until smooth. Add ricotta cheese and remaining filling ingredients and process again briefly.
Pour into the pastry base and bake 30 minutes at 180°C, or until set. Serve with Mock Cream (page 133) if desired. Serves 8.

♥ approx. 1·25g fat per serve

Tropical Custard Pie

base:
1 cup Nutrigrain
1/4 cup cornflake crumbs
1 1/2 tbspns apple juice concentrate*

filling:
1 x 415g can fruit salad in natural juice
1 x 400g can crushed pineapple, in natural juice
1/2 cup custard powder
2 tbspns low-joule berry jam (eg Cottee's)
1 tbspn lemon juice

Process the Nutrigrain in a food processor until it is crumbly. Add the cornflake crumbs and apple juice concentrate and process again until it resembles a wet breadcrumb texture. Press into a 28 cm round pie plate lined with plastic wrap to form a firm base and place in a freezer until the filling is ready.
In a saucepan, place canned fruits and their juice with the remaining filling ingredients. Blend custard powder into liquid thoroughly. Heat until almost boiling and the mixture thickens and coats the back of the spoon. Pour into prepared base and refrigerate to set.
Serve with Cherry Rum Liqueur Cream (page 134) if desired. Serves 8.

♥ approx. ·5g fat per serve

Mini Coconut Chocolate Tarts

You will need a 12 cup non-stick mini muffin tray for this recipe.

tart cases:
3 egg whites or substitute*, beaten
1/2 cup sugar or Splenda
1 tspn coconut essence
1 cup + 2 tbspns oat bran

filling:
1 tbspn custard powder
1 tbspn cocoa powder
3/4 cup skim milk
1/4 cup diet chocolate topping (Cottee's)
2 sachets powdered artificial sweetener or 1 tbspn sugar or Splenda

Preheat oven to 180°C.
Combine all the tart case ingredients in a bowl and mix thoroughly.
With wet fingers or the back of a firm plastic spoon, press the mixture into the muffin tins covering base and up the sides to form a cup-shaped outer shell.
Bake 8 minutes. Cool in tray for 5 minutes, then cool completely on a cake rack.
Meanwhile, make the filling.
Combine custard powder and cocoa powder in a small saucepan.
Slowly add milk and whisk to ensure thoroughly combined.
Add topping and stirring constantly, cook over medium heat to slowly bring mixture to a boil, until it boils and thickens. Remove immediately and stir through sweetener powder. Let stand 5 minutes then spoon into cases. Refrigerate.

♥ approx. 1·5g fat per tart

Creamy Apricot Flan

base:
1 1/4 cups Nutrigrain
1/3 cup cornflake crumbs
2 tbspns sugar or Splenda
2 egg whites or substitute*

filling:
1/2 cup low-fat cottage cheese
1 cup diet vanilla yoghurt
1 x 125g tub light Fruche apricot & honey flavour
1/2 cup sugar or Splenda
1 tspn grated orange rind
1 x 415g can pie apricots

Preheat oven to 180°C. Spray a 23cm pie plate with non-stick spray.
Process Nutrigrain in a food processor until it is crumbly. Add cornflakes
and Splenda and process briefly. Add egg whites and process again until
mixture is combined. Remove from processor and press evenly into pie
plate. Bake 7 minutes.
Beat cottage cheese, Fruche and sugar or Splenda. Add orange rind and
beat again.
Fold yoghurt through and spread into prepared base. Gently spread fruit
over top and refrigerate 2 hours.
Serve with Sweet Whipped Ricotta Cream (page 134) if desired.
Serves 8.

♥ approx. 1g fat per serve

Living Lite

sauces, toppings & basics

Apple Puree

Pureed fruit, particularly apple, is a fantastic substitute for fat (one for one) in baking muffins, cakes and other baked goods as it gives similar texture and lightness as oils and butter, without the fat and calories. You can use the jars of applesauce available in supermarkets, but I have not been able to find one that does not contain added sugar. I find it easier and healthier to make my own. I blend or process a couple of tins at one time and freeze 1/4 or 1/2 cup portions in small plastic bags. They can then be defrosted in the microwave as required.

2 x 800g cans pie apples (Mountain Maid or Ardmona)
1 tspn cinnamon (optional)

Process batches in a food processor. Measure out 1/4 or 1/2 cup portions and place in small plastic bags. Freeze and defrost as required.

Oil-Water Spray

You will require a clean plastic spray-misting bottle (the type sold in gardening department) to make this. If dollars permit, buy a stainless steel oil spray bottle (around $40) as they spray a more reliable and even spray.

Depending on the size of your bottle, measure 1 part oil to 7 parts water and fill bottle (eg. 2mls oil to 14mls water)

Obviously, you will need to shake the bottle before every use, as water and oil do not mix well. This spray is used for sauteing and stir-frying in some of the recipes in this book. Make a separate one for olive oil, sesame oil, peanut and canola oil if you wish.

Slimmer Sour Cream

1 cup low-fat ricotta cheese
1 cup plain non-fat yoghurt
1 tbspn lemon juice
freshly ground black pepper
pinch salt

Combine ingredients thoroughly in a food processor. Keep refrigerated.
♥ approx. ·5g fat per tbspn

Yoghurt Mint Sauce

1 cup plain non-fat yoghurt
3 tspns chopped fresh mint
1/4 tspn ground cumin powder
salt & pepper

Combine all ingredients thoroughly. Serve with fish or vegetable burgers.
Keep in refrigerator.
♥ neg. fat per tbspn

Fat-Free Mayonnaise

1 x 400g can condensed skim milk
1 tspn dry mustard
1 cup white vinegar

Combine thoroughly in a jar and keep refrigerated.
♥ neg. fat per tbspn

Mock Cream

1 cup low-fat ricotta cheese
2/3 cup plain non-fat yoghurt
1 tspn vanilla essence

Combine all ingredients and blend thoroughly in food processor.
♥ approx. ·5g fat per tbspn

Slim Whip

1 cup chilled skim milk
3 tspns skim milk powder
1 tspn vanilla essence
1 tspn sugar or Splenda

Whip or beat all the ingredients in a bowl until thick and creamy.
♥ neg. fat per tbspn

Sweet Maple Cinnamon Sauce

1 cup plain non-fat yoghurt
2 tbspns maple syrup
1/2 tspn vanilla essence
1/2 tspn cinnamon
2 tspns water

Blend all ingredients together and serve over desserts or cakes.
♥ neg. fat per tbspn

Cherry Brandy Liqueur Cream

1 cup low-fat cottage cheese
1 tbspn Splenda
2 tspns cherry brandy liqueur essence (Queen's brand)

Process all ingredients in food processor until smooth and thoroughly blended.
♥ approx. ·7g fat per tbspn

Citrus Cream

1 cup low-fat cottage cheese
2 1/2 tbspns sugar or Splenda
1 1/2 tspns freshly grated lemon rind
1 tspn vanilla essence

Process all ingredients in food processor until smooth and thoroughly blended.
♥ approx. ·7g fat per tbspn

Sweet Whipped Ricotta Cream

*I don't pretend that this version tastes just like whipped cream, but it is a great substitute to real cream (which is **very** high in fat).*

1 cup low-fat ricotta cheese
1 tbspn maple syrup or honey (or few drops of liquid sweetener)
1/4 – 1/2 cup skim milk (add to produce desired consistency)

Process all ingredients in food processor until smooth and thoroughly blended.
♥ approx. ·7g fat per tbspn

Chocolate Sauce

2 tbspns cocoa powder
3 tspns cornflour
2 tbspns sugar or Splenda
2 cups skim milk

Place dry ingredients in a small saucepan and combine thoroughly.
Blend a little milk into the dry ingredients, and mix ensuring no lumps
remain.
Add remaining milk and slowly bring mixture to a boil, stirring
constantly until it boils and thickens.
♥ neg. fat per tbspn

Baking Glaze

2 tbspns boiling water
1 tspn gelatine
2 tbspns jam

Combine and let cool slightly. Brush on as required.
♥ nil fat per tbspn

Guilt-Free Coconut Milk

1 x 375ml can evaporated low-fat milk
1 1/2 tspns coconut essence
1 1/2 tspns cornflour

Combine thoroughly. Use as you would normal coconut milk.
♥ approx. 6g fat entire recipe

Chive & Lemon Sauce

juice 1/2 small lemon
grated rind 1/2 small lemon
1/2 cup white wine
1 tspn grated fresh ginger
salt & pepper to taste
2 tspns arrowroot combined with 1 tbspn water
2 tbspns chopped fresh chives

In a small saucepan, combine lemon juice, rind, wine, ginger, salt and pepper and simmer uncovered 6 minutes.
Add arrowroot mixture.
Stirring continuously, simmer until the sauce is thick and clear. Remove from heat and add chives.
Serve over fish, fishcakes, or hot vegetables.

♥ neg. fat entire recipe

Creamy Mustard Sauce

1/2 cup fat-free chicken stock
1/2 cup white wine
1 tbspn wholegrain mustard
1/4 cup plain non-fat yoghurt
1 tbspn chopped fresh chives

Bring stock, wine and mustard to a boil in a small saucepan. Reduce heat and simmer until the liquid has reduced by half.
Let cool for 10 minutes.
Stir through yoghurt and chives. Serve over chicken.

♥ neg. fat entire recipe

Seafood Sauce

3 tbspns plain non-fat yoghurt
3 tbspns tomato sauce
1 1/2 tbspns oil-free French dressing
Tabasco sauce to taste
salt and pepper to taste
pinch paprika

Combine all the ingredients thoroughly with a whisk.
Serve over any seafood or fish.

♥ neg. fat per tbspn

Fat-Free White Sauce

Use this sauce as a basis for other flavours. Add herbs, mustards etc. to vary the flavour. To make a cheese sauce, add a little grated low-fat cheese (eg Seven) and grated Parmesan cheese.

2 tbspns plain flour
1 cup skim milk
1/3 cup fat-free vegetable stock
pinch nutmeg
salt and freshly ground black pepper

In a small saucepan, combine flour and a little of the milk and stir to form a paste.
Gradually add remaining milk and the stock and ensure well combined.
Stir over medium heat until it simmers and thickens. Cook 1 minute.
Remove from heat; add nutmeg and salt and pepper to taste.

♥ neg. fat per tbspn

Yoghurt Cheese

2 cups plain non-fat yoghurt - it must have no gelatine added (check ingredients listing)

Line a colander or strainer with a double thickness of cheesecloth (muslin) and place colander over a bowl. Alternatively, use a large coffee filter bag placed in top of a coffee percolator.
Spoon yoghurt into colander or coffee bag and refrigerate 8 hours or overnight to drain. After draining, place in a suitable container and keep refrigerated. Use as required. Makes approximately 1 1/4 cups.

Herbed Yoghurt Cheese

2 cups plain non-fat yoghurt (no gelatine)
1 tspn mixed herbs
dry mustard powder or powdered horseradish to taste

Follow instructions as above. After draining, mix herbs and mustard or horseradish through yoghurt. Place in a suitable container and keep refrigerated.

Sweet Yoghurt Cheese

2 cups plain non-fat yoghurt (no gelatine)
1/4 cup sugar or Splenda
2 tspns vanilla essence

Combine yoghurt, sugar or Splenda and vanilla essence thoroughly and drain following instructions as above. After draining, place in a suitable container and keep refrigerated.

♥ approx. 1g fat in each entire recipe

Living Lite

Living Lite Hints & Tips
Living Lite Exercise
Glossary
Recipe Index

Living Lite Hints & Tips

♥ Serve bagels (authentic ones are made with no added fat) instead of fat filled croissants, bought muffins or doughnuts. The fat in 10 bagels equals the fat in one croissant. One bagel contains only 2.5 grams of fat - one croissant contains a whopping 17 grams of fat! And a bagel will fill you up long before the croissant does!

♥ Spread fat-free yoghurt cheese (page 138) on the bagels instead of butter and save 4 grams of fat per teaspoon.

♥ By just replacing 1 1/2 teaspoons of butter with 1 tablespoon of jam or marmalade on your toast every day for one year you could lose as much as 5 1/2 kilograms!

♥ Gradually switch from full cream milk to skim milk and you save 9.5 grams of fat in one cup.

♥ Trim the fat from bacon and save 9 grams of fat per rasher. Beware of rindless bacon – the rashers are made from even fattier pork so you don't save on anything.

♥ Replace a regular bacon rasher with reduced-fat bacon and you'll save up to 12 grams of fat and over 120 calories per slice.

♥ Select high-fibre cereals like Vita Brits, Weeties, Corn Flakes, or Special K and add dried fruit for extra sweetening instead of sugar or honey,

♥ While Muesli is considered a healthy choice, most mixes are very high in fat. Some can contain 7 grams of fat in one small serve.

♥ While avocadoes contain "good fats" just half of a medium avocado contains 13g fat!

♥ Avoid coconut – 1 cup of desiccated coconut contains 60g of fat! Likewise with coconut milk – 1 cup contains 32g fat!

♥ Serve pancakes with cinnamon and icing sugar instead of butter and maple syrup.

♥ Pour low-fat yoghurt over fresh fruit with a handful of crunchy cereal for a delicious breakfast.

♥ Begin your meal with a bowl of stock-based soup, preferably vegetable, as studies have shown that it can reduce a tendency to overeat during the meal. Or start with a green salad to cut your appetite for the rest of the meal.

♥ Make your own low-fat garlic bread by spraying Italian bread with a quick spray of cooking oil and sprinkling with granulated garlic or garlic powder and herbs. Grill under a griller.

♥ Removing the skin from chicken breast will cut the fat by up to two thirds.

♥ Coat skinless chicken and fish with plain non-fat yoghurt or pureed low-fat cottage cheese to act as an adhesive for seasonings or crumbs before cooking.

♥ Use minced chicken or turkey instead of beef in meat loaves and hamburgers.

♥ Substitute a chicken sausage for a pork sausage and save 5g fat.

♥ Cut meat and poultry into smaller pieces strips and serve with filling foods like potato, pasta or rice to reduce fat amount in each serve.

♥ Top pizza with lots of extra vegetables like mushrooms, capsicum, pineapple and tomato instead of meat or extra cheese.

♥ Make low-fat pasta sauces with fresh or canned tomatoes, onions, mushrooms, capsicum, herbs, spices and stock. Add carrot or sweet potato for a change.

♥ Cook sweet potatoes instead of white potatoes for a sweeter flavour and eliminate the desire for butter or sauce.

♥ Substitute 1 tablespoon of butter with 1 tablespoon 99% fat-free mayonnaise and save over 15g fat. (Whole egg mayonnaise contains up to 20g fat.)

♥ Load up your sandwiches with lettuce, cucumber, tomatoes, salad sprouts, grated carrot instead of meat and cheese.

♥ Try a blend of plain non-fat yoghurt, fresh herbs and soy sauce to taste instead of regular mayonnaise in salads.

♥ Use thick slices of bread in making sandwiches to make it more filling.

♥ Select low-fat cheeses (eg Seven) and save up to 6g fat per 30g serve.

♥ Select pretzels or baked corn chips (eg. Freedom Foods) over potato chips to satisfy a salty crunchy craving.

♥ Make your own fat-free "chips" by toasting or microwaving pitta bread.

♥ Munch on raw carrot, celery, broccoli and mushrooms and dip in salsa instead of cheese and crackers or nuts.

♥ Dip pretzels or pitta bread chips in fat-free salsa instead of creamy dips and save up to 6g fat per tablespoon.

♥ Choose 98% fat-free crispbread (eg Salada) over water crackers, which can quickly add up to 4 grams of fat in 4 crackers.

♥ Buy non-fat yoghurts. After a while you'll never notice the difference.

♥ Keep low-fat snacks like dried fruit in your bag, glove box and desk drawer so you don't need the vending machines and snack bars.

♥ If eating out request all sauces and dressings on the side.

♥ If you feel it may be a difficult to find a low-fat meal on the menu, phone ahead to request one.

♥ Vegetarian meals are not always the better option – a lot of vegetarian dishes make up for the meat by adding loads of cheese and oil.

♥ Steer away from garlic bread. One slice in a restaurant can cost you up to 9g fat. Request some plain bread instead.

♥ Order a tomato-based pasta sauce instead of a creamy sauce and save a huge 32 grams of fat per average serve.

♥ Don't select dine-out places with smorgasbords to reduce the temptation to overeat to get your money's worth.

♥ Limit your alcohol intake - it adds empty calories, increases your appetite and weakens your resolve to turn down high fat foods.

♥ Ask how your dish is to be prepared before you order. Butter is often added to innocently steamed vegetables or it is used to grill the chicken and fish. Ask to have it omitted.

♥ Order your salad without dressing and take your own fat-free dressing. Or order lemon slices to squeeze onto your salad or vegetables.

♥ Don't order a bowl of chips while waiting for your meal to come. One small serve can cost you 10g fat.

♥ Beware the Caesar salad – just a 1 cup serve usually contains around 26g fat and 380 calories!

♥ Avoid mayonnaise-drenched salads – whole egg mayonnaise contains up to 20g fat per tablespoon.

♥ Avoid fried and sautéed foods – order grilled, poached, steamed or baked.

♥ Order skim milk in cappuccinos and smoothies. These days most places have this option available.

♥ Avoid sugary soft drinks and rich desserts.

♥ Buy the ultra low-fat (99.9% fat-free) ice creams over the full fat one, but remember they contain a lot of sugar.

♥ Indicators of high fat are the oily layers you find on the bottom of a paper bags and cardboard boxes that contain cakes, pizzas, biscuits and pastries.

♥ Opt for low-fat frozen yoghurt or fruit sorbets instead of ice cream.

♥ Forget the nuts on your sundaes. A 1/4 cup of nuts can add up to 200 calories and up to 18 grams of fat.

♥ Skip the topping on your ice cream and add fresh fruit instead. (Low-fat ice cream of course!)

♥ Check the labels on reduced-fat biscuits. Most contain less fat but make up for it in sugar and some have more calories than their regular counterpart.

♥ Satisfy a sweet craving with low-fat liquorice, boiled sweets, jelly babies, jellybeans, gumdrops, marshmallows all of which contain virtually no fat.

♥ Make your own fat-free cakes from this book for an indulgence. A typical bought slice of Black Forest cake can contain 18g fat!

♥ Make your own apple pie with baked apples or homemade apple sauce and a low-fat pastry and eliminate loads of fat.

♥ Substitute low-fat evaporated milk for the cream in rich dishes like quiche, cream soups and sauces. Just add a little cornflour to prevent it from separating.

♥ Use a very short burst of vegetable cooking spray instead of butter or oil or use the Oil-water Spray idea on page 131.

♥ Make extra portions when cooking and freeze them for later for when you arrive home late and are tempted to order in pizza.

♥ Use fat-free chicken stock with a pinch of garlic powder instead of oil or butter to sauté chicken and vegetables.

Living Lite Exercise

There are no excuses – even 10 minutes a day is better than none at all.

Suggestions:

♥ Try to walk 30 minutes a day – even if it is broken up into 3 x 10 minute walks.

♥ Walk with a friend for company & motivation.

♥ Exercise while you are watching TV – sit-ups, marching on the spot, anything!

♥ Tone-up exercises while standing cleaning your teeth, waiting in a queue, at the stove or washing up

♥ Do something you enjoy – you don't have to slog it out at the gym if you hate it

♥ Find the best time of the day and stick to it.

♥ Remember - you will never regret doing it after you have.

Glossary:

Apple juice concentrate: Syrup made from apple juice boiled and reduced to a concentrate. Use as a sweetener, and excellent to bind crumbs to make fat-free piecrusts (instead of butter). Can be used as a baking glaze. It is 66% sugar (honey is 80% sugar). Available in most large supermarkets and health food stores.

Apple Puree: use a commercial applesauce or see page 131 to make your own sugar-free.

Besan flour: flour made from ground chickpeas with a nutty taste. Buy in health food stores. If unavailable, use cornflour.

Chinese cooking wine: Like dry sherry. Buy in Asian food stores and some supermarkets.

Crunchola: cereal made by *Norganic* with no added fat, salt or sugar. Available in supermarkets or health food stores. Good for a crumble topping, to give a crunchy texture to baked goods, or as a texture substitute for nuts.

Curry paste: Good fat-free brands – *Sakims, Trident* and *Orchid*.

Dry roasted chickpeas: Make an excellent nut substitute. Contain very little fat. Found in selected health food shops.

Egg substitute: *Egg-like* made by *Country Harvest* used to substitute whole eggs or egg whites. A powder you mix with water. I have had great success using it in every egg recipe I have ever made - quiches, pies, baking, even ice cream. Available in supermarkets and health food stores.

Fat-free fruit mince: Use *Blackwood Lane* brand. Found in the supermarket - other fruit mince products contain suet (a solid white fat extracted from around the kidneys of cattle!)

Fat Replacer: Product made by *Orgran,* Available in supermarkets and health food stores. I used it in the Anzac Biscuits recipe, but have not tried it in any other recipes.

Kaffir lime leaves: Available dried or fresh in some supermarkets or buy from Asian food stores.

Lemongrass powder: Dried ground lemongrass. I have only found this in Asian grocery stores.

Liquid Smoke: Bottled hickory flavoured liquid. Gives food a smoked flavour and aroma. Available from gourmet food stores.

Maple syrup: *Steeve* is a Canadian brand of light maple syrup now available that contains 50% less calories than traditional maple syrup. Use normal maple syrup if unavailable.

Mirin: Mildly sweet Japanese syrup or rice wine. 14% alcohol, it is used only for cooking. Buy in Asian grocery stores or large supermarkets. If unavailable, use sweet white wine.

Prepared horseradish: Prepared horseradish is grated horseradish usually preserved in vinegar. Can be found bottled in the supermarket. Don't buy the horseradish cream (full of fat).

Prune puree: Great substitute for fat in baking particularly in chocolate recipes. Can be bought in supermarket. Look for brands with no added sugar (eg *Prunex*) or you can make your own by processing 90mls water with 1-1/3 cups pitted prunes to form a paste. For smaller amounts, buy jars of baby food prunes.

Quark (low-fat): available in health food shops and some supermarkets. It is a very low-fat soft cheese ideal for cheesecakes and as a base for dips.

Rice syrup/corn syrup: I use these as a fat substitute as they give the same crisp result in baked goods as butter does. (eg. biscuits). Although both syrups are sweeteners the taste is very subtle. This makes them suitable for use in savoury recipes. I use *Pureharvest* rice syrup and *Karo* corn syrup. Both are available in most supermarkets.

Risoni: Also called orzo or riso, a rice-shaped pasta found in the pasta section of the supermarket.

Splenda: I have found that this product used "spoon for spoon" is fabulous. It is expensive, but if cutting calories are important to you and you don't mind using an artificial sweetener, use it. I like it because it is made from sugar and suitable for baking. Use real sugar if you wish or use half sugar half Splenda.

Stevia liquid: Made from stevioside, a natural herb sweetener with no calories. As it is hundreds of times sweeter than sugar, use very sparingly – 1 tspn is equivalent to 1 cup sugar. Can be used for baking unlike many artificial sweeteners, as it is heat stable to 200°C.

Sumac: Made from berries from a native Turkish shrub and used widely in Middle Eastern cooking. Available from gourmet shops and food specialty stores.

Sun-dried tomatoes: Available in fruit & vegetable section of supermarket and health food stores. They are not packed in oil, just loose dried tomato halves. Reconstitute by placing in hot water or by adding to dishes at beginning of cooking.

Verjuice: made from unripened white grapes. I find it great to sauté in. It doesn't mask flavours, as it is non-acidic tasting. Maggie Beer has the most widely available product, and I find it in my local supermarket. Most gourmet food stores carry it.

Wasabi powder/paste: Japanese horseradish. Very hot. Available in the Asian section of supermarkets and in Asian food stores.

Recipe Index

Living Lite 2 is already under way!
If you would like prior notification of the *Living Lite 2* release date,
please complete (or photocopy and complete) the following form and
forward to the address below.

☐   Please notify me prior to the release of Living Lite 2

Name:

Address:

Phone: Fax:

Email:

Comments:

Please forward this form to:

LIVING LITE 2
Cut & Paste Studio Pty Ltd
39 First Avenue, Bridgewater SA 5155
Telephone: (08) 8339 4536   Facsimile: (08) 8339 8224

You will be notified by post when *Living Lite 2* is to be released.

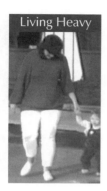

Living Heavy

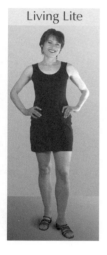

Living Lite

Are *you* Living Lite today?

Living Lite

Ultra Low-Fat & Fat-Free Recipes

Sandy Frazer

To order Living Lite

Please send me _____ copies of **Living Lite**
at $27.50 per book + $5.00 shipping
(Please add $2.50 per book thereafter)

Name : _____

Telephone : (   ) _____

Fax : (   ) _____

Email : _____

Delivery Address : _____

_____

_____ P/C _____

_____ Books @ 27.50 : $ _____

+ Shipping : $ _____

Total cost of purchase : $ _____

Method of payment :   Cheque/Money Order ☐
                 (Made payable to Cut & Paste Studio)

                Bankcard ☐

                VISA ☐

                MasterCard ☐

                Card Verification code _____
                (effective 4/01)

Cardholder Name : _____

Credit Card No : _____

Signature* : _____

Expiry Date : _____

*Please check credit card no. & expiry date before signing

Send to :   Cut & Paste Studio
           39 First Avenue
           Bridgewater S.A 5155

or fax to :   (08) 8339 8224

or Email your order with
full Credit Card details to :   lite@looksmart.com.au